DATE			

D1417826

The
Impaired
Physician

The Impaired Physician

Edited by

Stephen C. Scheiber

University of Arizona
Health Sciences Center
Tucson, Arizona

and

Brian B. Doyle

George Washington University
School of Medicine and Health Sciences
Washington, D.C.

Plenum Medical Book Company
New York and London

Library of Congress Cataloging in Publication Data

Main entry under title:

The Impaired physician.

Bibliography: p.
Includes index.
1. Physicians—Mental Health. I. Scheiber, Stephen C. II. Doyle, Brian B.,
1941 —   [DNLM: 1. Physicians—Psychology. 2. Physician impairment.
W 21 I34]
RC451.4.P5I46 1983   616.89′008861   82-22296
ISBN 0-306-41081-8

© 1983 Plenum Publishing Corporation
233 Spring Street, New York, N.Y. 10013

Plenum Medical Book Company is an imprint of
Plenum Publishing Corporation

Printed in the United States of America

TO
OUR FAMILIES

Contributors

JOLENE K. BERG, M.D., Family Practice Resident, St. John's Hospital, Department of Family Practice and Community Health, University of Minnesota Medical School, Minneapolis, Minnesota

DAVID W. CLINE, M.D., Associate Professor, Department of Psychiatry, University of Minnesota Medical School, and Coordinator of Medical Education, North Central Regional Medical Education Center, Minneapolis, Minnesota

BRIAN B. DOYLE, M.D., Associate Professor, Department of Psychiatry and Behavioral Sciences, George Washington University School of Medicine and Health Sciences, Washington, D.C.

JUDITH GARRARD, Ph.D., Associate Professor, Department of Psychiatry, University of Minnesota Medical School, Minneapolis, Minnesota

IRA D. GLICK, M.D., Professor, Department of Psychiatry, Cornell University Medical College, New York Hospital–Cornell Medical Center, New York, New York

DONALD LANGSLEY, M.D., Executive Vice-President, American Board of Medical Specialists and Immediate Past-President of American Psychiatric Association, Evanston, Illinois

CAROL C. NADELSON, M.D., Professor, Department of Psychiatry, Tufts University School of Medicine, Tufts–New England Medical Center, Boston, Massachusetts

MALKAH T. NOTMAN, M.D., Clinical Professor, Department of Psychiatry, Tufts University School of Medicine, Tufts-New England Medical Center, Boston, Massachusetts

DAVID W. PREVEN, M.D., Associate Professor, Department of Psychiatry, Albert Einstein College of Medicine of Yeshiva University, New York, New York

CAROLYN B. ROBINOWITZ, M.D., Clinical Professor, Department of Psychiatry and Behavioral Sciences, George Washington University School of Medicine and Health Sciences, and Deputy Medical Director of the American Psychiatric Association, Washington, D.C.

STEPHEN C. SCHEIBER, M.D., Professor, Department of Psychiatry, University of Arizona College of Medicine, Arizona Health Sciences Center, Tucson, Arizona

THOMAS G. WEBSTER, M.D., Professor, Department of Psychiatry and Behavioral Sciences and Department of Child Health and Development, George Washington University School of Medicine and Health Sciences, Washington, D.C.

Foreword

The Oath of Hippocrates, administered to generations of physicians as they embark on their profession, begins: "I will look upon him who shall have taught me this art even as one of my parents. I will share my substance with him, and I will supply his necessities, if he be in need." Despite that solemn promise, we have too often ignored or neglected the physician in trouble. Even if we could put aside the human concerns of one physician for an impaired colleague (can our profession truly permit that?), we must concede that our society can ill afford it. This book, which has been assembled and edited by Stephen C. Scheiber and Brian B. Doyle, may be a lifesaver for the doctor in trouble and will be a health-saver for the population of our country. A land which decried the lack of physicians a quarter century ago and spent the vast resources to double the number of graduates in medicine, cannot permit a tenth of all doctors to be out of commission. That would be a large, and for the most part preventable, addition to the cost of health care in America.

In this book, Scheiber and Doyle have gathered the expertise of many psychiatrists who are knowledgeable about the impaired physician. They have described the extent of the problem, have proposed ways to treat and even prevent impairment typical of a physician, have outlined the efforts of medical groups to deal with it, and have pointed out some of the special problems of women in medicine, and of families of physicians. The special focus on prevention as well as treatment will make this volume of special interest to educators in medical schools and hospitals.

We might ask why psychiatry has this special interest in the impaired physician. The reason is that most of the problems causing such impairment are psychiatric. The serious concerns are drugs, alcohol, depression, and marital problems. For the obvious physical problem, the physician will seek treatment more promptly. Here, too, the physician's conviction that he cannot get sick or that he should treat himself or that he doesn't want to bother his colleagues will make him delay. With mental disorder, the age-old stigma makes it even more difficult to admit that a problem exists and to seek appropriate help. It's easier to conceal a drinking or drug problem or to cover the personal pain of a depressive illness than to conceal a marked physical impairment. Though colleagues may suspect or recognize it, they are loathe to do something about it. Colleagues are troubled by the usual prohibitions against "tattling," by the complexities of overidentification with a fellow physician, and the fear that "There, but for the grace of God . . ." which generally conceals a countertransference problem. In this volume Scheiber and Doyle have highlighted the ways in which psychiatrists can make a major contribution to the recognition, treatment, and prevention of the disorders which impair physicians. These matters are the concerns of psychiatry. While we psychiatrists should take a leadership role in helping our psychiatric and nonpsychiatric colleagues who are in trouble, we cannot do it alone. The responsibility belongs to all of medicine, not just to one specialty.

Medicine may involve a high-risk career, but the rewards to society and to the physician have made it one of the most respected professions. We have the tools and the knowledge to reduce, alleviate, and perhaps even prevent some of the risks. To do so would benefit our citizens as well as our colleagues and their families. Scheiber, Doyle, and their contributors have shown us some of the ways and identified the problems yet to be solved.

DONALD LANGSLEY

Evanston, Illinois

Preface

"Physician, heal thyself!" The injunction has carried across the centuries, a reminder that those who would heal others had best look to their own health. Being an effective physician requires self-confidence and skill, for the demands of clinical practice are great. Many patients want to feel that their physicians are larger than life; this confidence in their physicians' strength sustains them and can help them get well. It is difficult for physicians to acknowledge their own human frailty while bearing appropriately their patients' needs that they be extraordinary. When the doctor is ill there are consequences for many others. This is particularly true when the physician has serious emotional difficulties. "The impaired physician" is a phrase which has come to denote doctors with psychiatric illness, alcoholism and/or abuse of other drugs, and suicide. This volume describes physicians with these difficulties.

The book results from the work of a group of psychiatrists who have longstanding interests in medical education and in clinical practice. Under the aegis of the Association for Academic Psychiatry (AAP), an organization of psychiatric teachers, we have written papers for and made presentations at local and national meetings of the American Psychiatric Association and the Association of American Medical Colleges. From the articles produced in the last five years, the co-editors have selected and included several in this book. We hope to reach a wider audience among doctors, where the subject of physician impairment has received increasing attention. We would like to reach nonmedical readers as well, because the problems of impaired physicians affect many lay people. Further, many other professional persons with responsible and important positions are subject to pressures similar to those experienced by physicians. Our observations, studies, and recommendations, while focused on medical students and physicians, can be more generally applied usefully to other persons as well.

Of the book's six parts, the first defines the nature and scope of the problem. In Chapter 1, "Emotional Problems of Physicians: Nature and Extent of Problems," Scheiber, while emphasizing some of the inadequacies of current data, estimates the extent of alcoholism, drug dependence, and other mental disorders in physicians. He raises the issue of physician suicide, and notes that physicians may have more than their share of troubled marriages. Scheiber outlines the signs and symptoms of the impaired physician, with overwork, increasing isolation, and depression as common themes. The diagnosable syndromes are end stages in the process. Throughout his course of disability, characteristically the impaired physician fails to ask for help.

In Chapter 2, Nadelson and Notman answer the question "What Is Different for Women Physicians?" While the number of women in medicine has risen dramatically in recent years, medical education and training has not accommodated to their special needs. That women find medical school and residency more psychologically stressful than do men is reflected in the higher rate of medical women who commit suicide during the training period. The divorce rate for female physicians is higher than that of male physicians, and is higher than that of the general population. Nadelson and Notman explore how different expectations of the women, both of themselves and by society, contribute to their greater burdens. Problems include the absence of satisfactory role models, negative attitudes toward women physicians, and conflicts between career and childbearing and childrearing. Medicine provides a satisfying way for men to gratify nurturant wishes while achieving high status and traditionally masculine goals. Women physicians have major conflicts concerning achievement and nurturance. Further, applicants to medical school tend to be higher achievers, and women appear to be more conflicted than men about issues of achievement and competition. Women physicians find that their roles proliferate, and when pressured to limit their professional aspirations they will more often do so than will their husbands. Nadelson and Notman specify institutional and educational changes that would improve the picture for women in medicine.

Problems of drug addiction and alcoholism among physicians are the subject of Chapter 3, by Webster. The risk of drug addiction for physicians is estimated to be 30–100 times that of the general population. While alcoholism among physicians is a serious problem, its rate is comparable to that of the lay population. With adequate treatment, however, the prognosis is relatively good for physicians dependent on alcohol or other drugs. As expected, there is a high incidence of other psychiatric diagnoses in the affected physicians. Although "work strain" is the most common presumed causal agent, substantial evidence exists for personality problems and difficulties long before medical school in many affected physicians. The medical profession locally and nationally is providing increasingly effective treatment and follow-up, but early identification and intervention is still problematic. Webster cites the

Georgia Disabled Doctors Program as one helpful model for early intervention. He concludes Chapter 3 with recommendations.

In Chapter, 4, Preven investigates the controversial subject of physician suicide. He asserts that statistics purporting to show a high rate of physician suicide are unfounded: there is no difference between the suicide rate for male physicians and age-matched men in the United States. While the suicide rate of women physicians is greater than that of nonphysician peers, it is similar to the rate of male physicians. A new study indicates that psychiatrists are overrepresented in the percentage of physician deaths due to suicide. Preven discusses difficulties in identifying and treating suicidal physicians. He emphasizes that special measures are necessary to cope with the impact of a physician's suicide, advocating a process in which survivors can deal with their feelings about the loss. A Physician's Mortality Study, recently sponsored by the American Medical Association and the American Psychiatric Association, performs psychological autopsies on physician suicides. The results may prove broadly beneficial.

Part II focuses on medical education as a natural setting for prevention, early identification, and treatment of physician impairment. In Chapter 5, Doyle and Cline review "Approaches to Prevention in Medical Education." They report that a survey of 20 medical schools for primary and secondary prevention of physician impairment has somewhat disappointing results. With specific and noteworthy exceptions, faculty at these medical schools provide little systematic attention to preventive measures. Faculty advisor systems work poorly; existing student-to-student advisor systems generate more enthusiasm. At over half the medical schools surveyed, there are small groups having psychological support as either an explicit or implicit purpose. At some schools, groups organized around special interests such as women's issues, minority students, etc., have supportive functions. A few schools use the orientation phase to identify possible sources of difficulty for students and to begin building support systems for them. Some measures for secondary prevention, making possible earlier diagnosis and prompt treatment, are controversial. For example, opinion is markedly divided about the appropriateness of psychiatric screening by admissions committees. At all schools, poor academic performance is a warning signal which gets prompt attention. How to detect or help the student who does well academically but not otherwise is problematic. Most of the schools give students abundant cognitive information about physician impairment; efforts to engage the students emotionally with the issues are less effective. Most faculty and staff surveyed feel that prompt, confidential help is available for troubled students. Chapter 5 also contains an example in which a Continuing Medical Education (CME) course is used for prevention. Doyle and Cline describe an educational experiment that provides unsolicited information about alcoholism and drug abuse to physicians enrolled in a CME course about pulmonary disease and hypertension. The preliminary results are encouraging, but much remains to be done.

In Chapter 6, "The Medical School Admissions Committee: A Preventive Psychiatry Challenge," Scheiber strongly advocates using the admissions process for screening. Problems evident long before medical school, and recognizable patterns of family difficulty characterize students who later become impaired physicians. Since admissions committees now tend to have unreliable and inconsistent subjective reports of students, committees must rely excessively on the results of aptitude tests and grade-point averages. In remedy, Scheiber proposes a comprehensive data base for assessing the psychological well-being of candidates, including psychiatric assessment of those identified as high-risk. He urges responsible use of these data to provide the necessary support to high-risk medical students. Over 20–30 years, he asserts, admissions committee members will be able to compare outcomes and determine how effective their preventive efforts have been.

Nadelson, Notman, and Preven finish this part of the book with Chapter 7, "Medical Student Stress, Adaptation, and Mental Health." Medical school is stressful for many reasons, with major intellectual demands being made of students trying to resolve major developmental issues of intimacy and identity. Data are generally unsatisfactory concerning the incidence of suicide, serious mental illness, and drug and alcohol abuse in medical students. Overall, 10%–25% of them seek psychiatric consultation or enter treatment, a proportion comparable to that in other graduate student populations. While poor academic work is often associated with emotional difficulty, a good record does not guarantee emotional well-being. The preclinical years are often particularly stressful, with perfectionist students having to accept their inability to master all of the course material. Nadelson, Notman, and Preven include case examples of student difficulties and various psychiatric interventions.

Part III has chapters devoted to support and treatment for the impaired physician. Glick, in Chapter 8, discusses "Family Therapy for the Impaired Physician." He asserts not only that the physician's impairment affects families, but also that family treatment can be more helpful than individual treatment. He illustrates his points by case examples from 10 consecutive physician-family referrals. He advocates fuller use of the family approach, with controlled-outcome studies still necessary to test its helpfulness.

In Chapter 9, Webster addresses "Psychotherapeutic Issues in Psychiatric Treatment of Physicians with Alcohol and Drug Abuse Problems." In the process of developing an early intervention, he emphasizes, there is a need for the psychiatrist to have a sense of comfortable acquaintance with the medical colleague in treatment. Ensuring privacy for the affected physician is highly desirable. The treating psychiatrist must develop genuine respect and warmth for the physician-patient, gradually building trust in the therapeutic relationship. It is useful to address drug and alcohol dependency as specific problems independent of associated psychodynamic factors. Webster agrees that involvement of the family in treatment is strongly indicated, but that this also requires clinical judgment, specific assessment, and management. He notes that a psychiatrist serving as an auxiliary conscience is more important in advanced stages of illness than in earlier phases. Recovered alcoholic and formerly drug-addicted physicians are often valuable adjuncts to successful treatment. Hospitalization can be useful, in addition to detoxification, for establishing the firm working relationships necessary for rehabilitation. The psychiatrist is responsible for overall case management, for working with the family and collaborating with professional colleagues. Always, Webster emphasizes, the treating psychiatrist provides hope to the patient and to the family.

Part IV addresses "Special Problems in Treating Physicians." In Chapter 10, Doyle writes about "Responsibility, Confidentiality, and the Psychiatrically Ill Physician." He notes numerous obstacles to disturbed physicians' seeking psychiatric help, as the affected doctor, family, and colleagues often collude to deny and avoid. The sick physician's symptoms threaten the equilibrium of his colleagues. Doyle includes recommendations for helping students as well as physicians to care for themselves and for each other.

In Chapter 11, Robinowitz attends to the myths and realities of "The Physician as a Patient." Health care for medical students and residents is often inadequate. The medical culture encourages physicians to suppress their own symptoms to serve others. Doctors are frequently astonished when they become ill because they see themselves as invulnerable. Once ill, doctors tend to insist on being treated as special patients, with serious consequences. Professional courtesy, while well-intentioned, may result in poorer treatment. There can be elaborate covert negotiations about who is in charge of treatment, with the physician patient usually reluctant to relinquish control.

Part V, "The Impaired Physician: A Collective Responsibility," consists of two chapters. In Chapter 12, "The Impaired Physician and Organized Medicine," discusses how organized medicine has responded at several levels to the needs of impaired physicians. The American Medical Association (AMA) has led actively with special national programs since 1975. In addition the AMA has a variety of other programs, including the development of model legislation concerning physician licensure. The American Medical Student Association and the American Psychiatric Association have each sponsored activities and programs relating to the impaired physician. Fifty state medical associations have authorized the formation of definitive programs. State committees usually rely on a team approach by concerned colleagues. Committee members work to ensure privacy and confidentiality, using coercive methods only to ensure the physician's compliance. Under some circumstances the sick physician can choose who will treat him while a committee-appointed monitor assesses whether the colleague involved can continue to practice. The state plans in Pennsylvania and California demonstrate the variety of effective approaches available. Methods vary for determining when the physician can practice. Followup is an important aspect of any program. Organized medicine is increasingly able to take care of its own when they are impaired.

In Chapter 13, Berg and Garrard write about "The Extent of Psychosocial Support of Residents in Family Practice Programs." Work demands of training programs frequently conflict with residents' personal needs and with their responsibilities to spouse, children, and household. Berg and Garrard have shown that programs in family practice and psychiatry are more likely to offer psychosocial support to their residents than are programs in other specialty areas. Among family practice programs, 3 of 11 kinds of support tend to occur together: seminars or speakers dealing with emotionally charged medical issues, seminars or speakers dealing with the stress and conflicts of being a physician, and finally, professional counselors. While family practice programs generally offer considerable psychosocial support to their residents, those which most support the family needs, such as family support groups, part-time residencies, and child-care services, are least available.

In the final part of the book, Appendix A lists the state programs for the impaired physician available, with the names and addresses of contact people in these states. This list, along with the American Medical Association Bibliography on the Impaired Physician in Appendix B, were provided by Emanuel Steindler of the Department of Mental Health, Division of Scientific Affairs of the American Medical Association.

Contents

   with Alcohol and Drug Abuse Problems 109
       THOMAS G. WEBSTER

IV. Special Problems in Treating Physicians

10. Responsibility, Confidentiality, and the Psychiatrically Ill
    Physician 125
        BRIAN B. DOYLE

11. The Physician as a Patient............................... 137
        CAROLYN B. ROBINOWITZ

V. The Impaired Physician: A Collective Responsibility

12. The Impaired Physician and Organized Medicine............ 147
        CAROLYN B. ROBINOWITZ

13. Residents in Family Practice: Psychosocial Support 157
        JOLENE K. BERG AND JUDITH GARRARD

VI. Recommendations

14. Conclusions and Recommendations........................ 169
        STEPHEN C. SCHEIBER AND BRIAN B. DOYLE

    Appendices 173

    Index 199

I

Emotional Problems of Physicians
What Are They?

1

Emotional Problems of Physicians
Nature and Extent of Problems

STEPHEN C. SCHEIBER

The life of a physician can be personally rewarding and professionally fulfilling. The physician is in a position to earn the respect of his peers, the admiration of his patients, and the love of his family. Frequently leaders in their community, physicians have a potential for personal and professional growth that is enormous. Most physicians prosper and live a rich, emotionally satisfying life. A minority of physicians, however, are emotionally troubled. This chapter discusses these emotional problems of physicians.

These emotional problems of physicians have not been well studied; they have been concealed and underreported, and have been poorly understood. The available studies reveal that the major problems are alcoholism and drug addiction, depression and suicide, and troubled marriages. The studies available rely on inpatient psychiatric admissions, psychiatric office practices, obituaries printed in the *Journal of the American Medical Association,* disciplinary actions of state boards of medical examiners, studies of medical student populations, and one prospective study. All studies suffer from the fallacies inherent in small samples, from attempts to generalize from limited data, and in most cases from poor controls.

METHODOLOGICAL PROBLEMS

The reasons for the lack of data are many. The study of emotionally disturbed physicians is painful. a'Brook et al. point out that the physi-

STEPHEN C. SCHEIBER • Department of Psychiatry, University of Arizona College of Medicine, Tucson, Arizona. Reprinted with permission from *Arizona Medicine,* vol. 34, May 1977.

cian-patient tends to deny patienthood.[1] He or she hides emotional syndromes from peers, family, and self.[2,3] For the physician to admit emotional problems raises the threat of economic loss. Where competency to practice as a physician is an issue or where addiction and self-prescriptions are known, then legal sanctions to limit or discontinue practice are threatening. Modlin points out that the emotional signs and symptoms are subtle and often insidious. They include the "secret drink, the surreptitious pill, and the private thought of suicide." There is frequently a conspiracy of silence between the physician-patient and his family and colleagues. The prepotent reason for concealing this problem is likely the "threat to the physician-patient's self-concept, self-image, and self-esteem."[4]

Medical colleagues fail to recognize or report the physician-patient for a variety of reasons or rationalizations. Colleagues frequently believe the myth, however false, that physician-patients ought to be able to take care of themselves. Hence, they do not make any overtures to help or to respond to the physician-patient's family's pleas for help. To report physician-patients as emotionally ill may be considered a betrayal and contribute to a suffering colleague's economic and legal difficulties. The lack of recognition of a physician-patient's distress is related to the colleague's conscious or unconscious denial that a physician can be emotionally disturbed. Further, it is likely related to the personal threat to his colleague of "There, but for the grace of God, go I."

EMOTIONAL PROBLEMS OF PHYSICIANS: RECOGNITION AND PREVALENCE

In spite of reporting difficulties, available figures suggest which are the leading emotional problems of physicians. Based on studies of disciplinary actions against physicians of three state boards of medical examiners, the identified impairments include alcoholism (2.3%–3.2% of registered physicians), drug dependence (0.9%–2.0%), and other mental disorders (0.9%–1.3%).[5] It is obvious that these figures are gross underestimates of these problems since medical examining boards become involved in only the most serious problems with the most overt behavioral deviations. The American Medical Association estimated that 7%–8% of doctors are now or will become alcoholics. Currently there are an estimated 10,000 alcoholic physicians.[6]

Suicide rates derived from data presented in the *Journal of the American Medical Association* point to more than 100 physician suicides a year, the equivalent of the size of an average graduating class of medical students.[7] Again, these figures underrepresent the true rates since they are dependent on other sources reporting the causes of death. In studying these statistics, Blachly et al. found that there were more deaths by suicide than by other violent means.[7] It is well known that many coroners conceal suicides by physicians by reporting only the presumed pathophysiological pathway, e.g., cardiac arrest or pulmonary failure. Rose and Rosow, in a careful computerized study in California of over 200,000 deaths, demonstrated that physicians and health-care workers are twice as suicide prone as the general population.[8]

Studies by Vaillant et al. reveal that 47% of physicians had bad marriages compared with 32% of the control sample.[9] Evans studied 50 wives of physicians, most of whom were hospitalized for depression[10]; 82% reported unsatisfactory sexual relationships. The absent husband was viewed as a significant precipitating factor in the depression of these wives.

EMOTIONAL PROBLEMS—DRUG ADDICTION

Over 4000 physicians in the United States, or 1.5% of practicing doctors, are known addicts. Estimates range from 30 to 100 times the rate of the general population[11]: 15% of known addicts are physicians; 15% are registered nurses and pharmacists. In one psychiatric inpatient study 27% of physicians were admitted for drug addiction, 30% for alcoholism, and 43% for other psychiatric disorders.[12] Another study revealed that 43 of 93 psychiatric admissions of physicians were for drug- or alcohol-addiction problems.[13] Unlike other addicts, the average age of onset in physicians is 40. Sedatives, tranquilizers, and stimulants are more commonly abused agents than narcotics.

Modlin and Montes's studies have shown that the common rationalizations for drug abuse are overwork, fatigue, and physical illness.[11] However, they demonstrated that the key factors are the predisposing personality of the physician and the easy availability of drugs. The complaints of overwork are often related to an inability to say "no" to patients, to referrals, to committee assignments, or to community obligations. These addiction-prone physicians have no outlets for their pent-up frustrations. Fatigability is usually related to the lack of satisfying marital and family relationships, lack of satisfying participation in community affairs, lack of recreation and avocations, and an underlying neurotic conflict about medical practice. Physical illnesses most often include psychosomatic ones: ulcers, asthma, hypertension, colitis, migraine headaches, and arthritis.

Modlin and Montes's studies[11] of addicted physicians show that only 3% held their fathers in esteem and only 13% felt warmth toward their mothers. They were sickly as children, having had disorders such as colic, enuresis, and other systemic illnesses; they tended to be compliant youths. More than 50% had alcoholic fathers. And 75% have unsatisfactory marital relationships.

Nine percent of physician addicts commit suicide.[14]

DEPRESSION AND SUICIDE

Pitts et al. estimated the prevalence of affective disorders among medical students at 7.5%.[15] Sainsbury estimates that 50% of persons committing suicide suffered from an affective disorder.[16]

Some personality traits of the "good doctor," including obsessionality, lack of pleasure seeking, and feelings of indispensibility, lend themselves to depression. With declining energies of middle life and the subsequent inability to maintain the pace of the "good doctor," the vulnerable physician is prone to depression. As in other populations, depression in physicians is a treatable illness.[17]

The studies of suicide in physicians reveal that the rate of male physicians is 1.15 times greater than the expected rate of the male population. For female physicians the rate is 3 times greater than expected. In the age group over 45, there is a marked excess in expected rate. Steppacher and Mausner's study of the *Journal of the American Medical Association* obituaries revealed that 12 of the 40 suicides in women occurred during training.[18] In the 25–39 age group, 26% of all physician deaths are attributed to suicide.[19] Many "accidental" deaths, such as one-car accidents, solo-flight airplane accidents, and drownings, are suicides, but are not recognized or reported as such. The most common cause of physician suicide is the ignoring of or failure to recognize depression.[20] Suicide prevention is urgently needed among physicians.[21]

TROUBLED MARRIAGES

The controlled study by Vaillant and colleagues documented that 47% of physicians have bad marriages.[9] Modlin and Montes's studies of physician addicts shows that 75% of them have difficulties with sexual relations.[11] Evans studied physicians' wives who were emotionally ill, mostly with depression. Of 50 patients, 16 presented with drug overdoses; 9 of the 16 were given the drugs by their physician husbands.[10] Duffy's review of physicians' wives admitted for psychiatric hospitalizations revealed almost half of 107 studied were abusing medications. Barbiturates were the most common drugs of abuse, but narcotics and stimulants were also overused.[22] This pattern is similar to that of the physician addict.

The average age of onset of depression in Evans's study of physicians' wives was 40. This again corresponds with the age when physicians become emotionally ill. If the sick physician turns to his wife for initial help and she is depressed, then she will not, and often cannot, be of help. Since her depression is often precipitated by feelings of abandonment based on being left alone by her husband in the early years of marriage, she may not only not hear her physician husband's cry for help, but may be outright rejecting.

The medical couples who have been studied are almost exclusively physicians and their wives. With the increasing number of female medical students, many of whom marry and have children, studies are now being conducted to examine the special issues of the woman physician and her marriage.[23,24] Nadelson and Notman in Chapter 2 on women and medicine address some of the special problems of two-career marriages.

Glick describes approaches to treating the physician's family in Chapter 8, on family therapy.

SIGNS AND SYMPTOMS

Waring describes the pattern of progression of signs and symptoms of a physician in distress.[2] The key is a chaotic life. The distressed physician will often start irregular office hours, be prone to poor eating and sleeping habits, and will be inefficient and disordered in his work. He becomes tense, insecure, and unsure of himself. Difficult patients with difficult problems especially aggravate his tension. He fails to request consultation with colleagues for fear of losing face. Self-medication with alcohol or drugs, or both, may temporarily ameliorate the symptoms.

He may seek relief at home, only to be rejected. This may lead to his burying himself in his office with increasing office hours, and an increasing need to feel indispensible. Alternatively, he may neglect his practice. He lacks outside interests and recreational pursuits, With fewer assets and energy to deal with his problems, he may then try to ward off his depression in varied ways. These include extramarital affairs (sometimes with patients), excessive spending on luxuries, gambling on high-risk stocks or real estate (in the name of investment), or plunging impulsively into youthful endeavors, such as vigorous athletic activities for which he has inadequate training and tolerance.

When these attempts fail, fatigue, tension, and depression follow. Drug abuse increases. Irritability with patients reflects the physician's feeling that all he does is give, with no reciprocity on the patient's part.

Depression, drug addiction, termination of marriages, and suicide are end stages in the process. Throughout, characteristically the emotionally disturbed physician fails to ask for help.

DISCUSSION

The statistics available regarding emotionally ill physicians represent the tip of the iceberg. Suicide rates as reported in the *Journal of the American Medical Association* are underrepresented. Alcoholism and addiction rates are gleaned from disciplinary actions of state medical examination boards or estimated by the American Medical Association. Behavioral manifestations of the problems must be so gross as to lead to a major public complaint, subsequent investigations, and then action. The subtler, better concealed manifestations in other disturbed physicians go unchecked, unreported, and untreated. Malfunctioning marriages of physicians have been studied mostly on the basis of inpatient admissions. This sample again represents only the most severe of the existing problems.

The traditional medical student has been described as overly ambitious, upwardly mobile, highly competitive, and obsessional in his studies without allowing for a diversity of interests. Also, the traditional physician has worked long hours and has been in solo practice, with no relief for night call and nobody accessible for immediate consultation. He frequently was found in short supply in underpopulated areas.

With the predicted surfeit of physicians in the future, and the current oversupply of some specialists in urban centers, the practice of medicine may very well become an eight-hour work day. This may remove some of the pressures of excessive time spent in pursuit of one's profession. Students may no longer be selected for their highly competitive characteristics, but may be persons with multiple interests whose life goals may not include medicine as the highest priority. They will be joining group practices with adequate coverage for night call. Many more physicians will accept salaried positions with fixed hours and fixed incomes. With a surfeit of doctors, physicians may have abundant time to become artists, spend weekends in family-oriented activities, and find fulfillment in areas outside of medicine. There may be a shift in the character of the physician, from an overly obsessional male physician to a more nurturing female physician. All these factors will allow the delivery of physicians' services to become more flexible.

These descriptions about the future of the practice of medicine and the character and lifestyle of physicians are purely speculative. In the meantime, studies need to continue to focus on areas of impairment. Further studies are required of the troubled life of a minority of physicians who are impaired.

REFERENCES

1. a'Brook MF, Hailstone JD, McLaughlin EJ: Psychiatric illness in the medical profession. *Br J Psychiat* 113:1013–1023, 1967.
2. Waring EM: Psychiatric illness in physicians: A review. *Compr Psychiat* 15:519–530, 1974.
3. Ross J: The physician as psychiatric patient: A few special problems. *Psychiatr Digest* 36–46, 1971.
4. Modlin H: The disabled physician. *J Kans Med Soc* 76:295–297, 324, 1975.
5. AMA Council on Mental Health: The sick physician: Impairment by psychiatric disorders, including alcoholism and drug dependence. *JAMA* 223:684–687, 1973.
6. Steindler EM: *The Impaired Physician.* Chicago, American Medical Association, 1975, p 7.
7. Blachly PH, Disher W, Roduner G: Suicide by physicians. *Bull Suicidology,* December 1968, pp 1–18.
8. Rose KD, Rosow I: Physicians who kill themselves. *Arch Gen Psychiat* 29:800–805, 1973.
9. Vaillant GE, Sobowale NC, McArthur C: Some psychological vulnerabilities of physicians. *N. Engl J Med* 287:372–375, 1972.
10. Evans JL: Psychiatric illness in the physician's wife. *Am J. Psychiat* 122:159–163, 1965.
11. Modlin HC, Montes A: Narcotic addiction in physicians. *Am J Psychiat* 121:358–365, 1964.
12. Vincent MO, Robinson EA, Latt L: Physicians as patients: Private psychiatric hospital experience. *Can Med Assoc J* 100:403–412, 1969.
13. Duffy, JC, Litin EM: Psychiatric morbidity of physicians. *JAMA* 189:982–992, 1964.
14. Putnam PL, Ellinwood EH: Narcotic addiction among physicians: A two year follow-up. *Am J Psychiat* 122:745–748, 1966.
15. Pitts FN, Jr, Winokur G, Steward MA: Psychiatric syndromes, anxiety symptoms and response to stress in medical students. *Am J Psychiat* 118:333–340, 1961.
16. Sainsbury P: Suicide and depression, in Coppen AJ, Walk A(eds): *Recent Developments in Affective Disorders.* London, Headley Brothers, 1968, pp 1–13.
17. Bittker TE: Reaching out to the depressed physician. *JAMA* 236:1713–1716, 1976.
18. Steppacher R, Mausner J: Suicide in male and female physicians. *JAMA* 228:323–328, 1974.
19. DeSole D, Aaronson S, Singer P: Suicide and role strain among physicians. Paper presented to APA, Detroit, May, 1967.
20. Freeman W: Psychiatrists who kill themselves. *Am J Psychiat* 124:846–847, 1967.
21. Kosbab P: Suicide prevention in physicians. *New Physician* 21:21–23, 1972.

22. Duffy JC: *Emotional Issues in the Lives of Physicians.* Springfield, Ill, Charles C Thomas, 1970, p 23.
23. Eisenberg L: The distaff of Aesculapius—the married woman as physician. *JAMWA* 33:84–88, 1981.
24. Johnson FA, Johnson CL: Role strain in high commitment career women. *J Am Acad Psychoanal* 4:13–36, 1976.

2

What Is Different for Women Physicians?

CAROL C. NADELSON AND MALKAH T. NOTMAN

In the past decade medical schools have admitted substantially greater numbers of women students. Currently, 26.5% of matriculated students are women, compared with 9% in 1968.[1] That women are no longer such a small minority and that their representation in the profession is continuing to increase are facts with far-reaching implications.

It is only within the last 5 years that there have been enough women in medicine to begin to consider collecting comparative data on their functioning and impairment, as well as on the stresses experienced by both male and female physicians. While there is a body of literature on alcoholism, drug addiction, and other symptoms of male physicians, the literature contains almost no data on these problems for women.[2] Either the data are not broken down between men and women, or the numbers of women in the samples are extremely small and therefore it is difficult to generalize.[3,4] Thus to arrive at an assessment of the situation one must rely on limited data; on inferences from students or other women professionals, or both; and on clinical reports.

The effort to enable a significant number of women to gain access to medical careers has been fruitful, but it also presents a dilemma. While intending to be helpful, it is possible to perform an inadvertent disservice by presenting women as particularly vulnerable. A potential conflict of loyalties exists between the responsibility toward an individual or group and the obligation to the profession and the public. The confidentiality necessary to protect and support the individual and to prevent stigmatizing or labeling at times interferes with the exercise of responsibility to uncover and understand problems.

CAROL C. NADELSON • Department of Psychiatry, Tufts University School of Medicine, Boston, Massachusetts   MALKAH T. NOTMAN • Department of Psychiatry, Tufts University School of Medicine, Boston, Massachusetts.

This dilemma dissolves to some extent when one examines the actual nature of the stresses and their sources. Many of the problems of women in medicine in the past can be considered to have derived from their isolation as a minority group, with all the implications of that status. Now that women comprise over 10% of physicians, there is less isolation. However, many women still report that there is little attention to specific needs, such as pregnancy. Thus the difficulties women face continue to relate in part to the rigidities of medical training and practice.

Identifying problems can lead to potential solutions, rather than to exclusion. Many of the constraints are also applicable to male physicians, who often lead lives which do not permit time for families or other interests. Concerns about the needs of women consequently enable us to focus on problems which are universal for all physicians.

DO THE STRESSES FOR MEN AND WOMEN DIFFER?

Evidence collected before the increase in numbers of women in medicine indicates that they have had a different and probably more stressful psychological experience than men. Phelps in 1968[5] reported that medical school dropout rates for male and female students for academic reasons were similar. However, of those leaving for non-academic reasons (usually personal), 8% were women and 3% were men. This gap is closing, and the difference in attrition between male and female medical students is now 1%.[6] Attrition rate, however, is only one indicator of stress and does not describe the entire experience.

Adsett[7] reported that a greater percentage of women medical students than men sought psychiatric counseling. He commented, however, that it was not clear if this is related to a greater ability to ask for help, or to the role conflicts or environmental pressures, which are greater for women. Since women in the United States generally use psychiatric facilities more than men, the same questions have been raised about this difference.[8] Weinberg and Rooney[9] cited "problems of adjustment," which they thought were especially related to the small numbers of women, as significant factors accounting for the lower academic achievement of the women in their study who were in the first year of medical school. It is important to note, however, that over the 4 years, academic achievement has not been different for men and women.

Evidence that problems continue to exist after medical school is found in the data of Steppacher and Mausner,[10] who reported that while the suicide rate for male physicians was 1.15 times that of the overall male population, the female physician rate was 3 times that expected for women. Furthermore, of the group of women who killed themselves, 40% were under age 40, while less than 20% of the males committed suicide prior to age 40. More suicides occurred among women than among men during the training period, and a substantial proportion of these women were single.

Another indicator which contributes to the view that there are greater stresses for women in medicine can be seen in the differential divorce rates for men and women physicians. While the divorce rate for male professionals, including physicians, is lower than that in the general population, the divorce rate for female physicians is higher than for male physicians and higher than the general population.[11] In dual-career couples in other occupations, as well as in medicine, the rate is higher than that for "traditional" couples. Since 80% of female physicians marry either physicians or other professionals, their marriages are vulnerable.[12] Further, since this lifestyle pattern is relatively new, there are few role models and little substantial in-depth data on marital adjustment and conflict.

Women physicians who do not marry professionals are also likely to have unstable marriages. Often their growth in status, relative to their husbands, puts a strain on the marriage. The discrepancies of interest and lifestyle, which might have been less discernable when both were younger, become a problem. The husband's expectations of a more conventional wife may come into conflict with the wife's aspirations, needs, or capacities.[13]

While data on divorce and suicide are dramatic, and other data on alcoholism, drug abuse, or rate of mental illness are indicative of impairment, they do not deal with the pain and distress which is reported clinically. These do not necessarily produce frank symptoms, or overt failure of performance, but they may reduce satisfaction and optimal functioning.

MEDICAL TRAINING: DEMANDS AND CONSEQUENCES

Medical education shares many characteristics with other graduate and professional training. There are, however, some specific and unique components which distinguish it from other fields. The length, rigidity, and intensity of demands from the beginning of medical school through residency is unparalleled in other professional or graduate programs. Although the same number of years may be required, the inflexible commitment of time and energy, and the responsibility demanded for medicine, is unique.

During this period a number of personal and educational goals must be accomplished: (1) the consolidation and integration of personal identity, and separation from family; (2) the acquisition of a large body of medical information; (3) the development of skills related to medical practice; (4) the development of a professional identity; and (5) the formulation and implementation of career and life goals.

The process of medical education occurs within a transitional developmental stage in the life of the student. During this time there must be a shift from a position of dependence on others, especially the family, toward the acquisition of greater personal independence and the capacity to assume major responsibilities for others.[14,15] This shift, concomitant with the enormous emotional, intellectual, and time demands, and constant exposure to crises in other people's lives, is a stressful experience in itself. It requires the development of new modes of adaptation.

Many students encounter real changes in their families at this time. Emotional crises, physical illness and death, separations and divorce, have a considerable impact.[16]

Women have been in a different position than men in that they "traditionally" have been expected to assume more of the direct caretaking responsibility for their own parents and those of their spouses, as they grow old and perhaps ill. Thus the demands on a woman student and physician may be greater when she is also burdened by the enormous drain of her medical training and practice. Since she cannot always perform optimally in each area, conflict, guilt, and anxiety may result.

Past adaptive and defensive styles may prove to be inadequate for the new situations encountered in medical school. Keniston[17] has described medical students' reliance on intellectual defense mechanisms, with reinforcement of isolation and repression of affect. The overemphasis on these mechanisms may restrict the individual's ability to respond in other ways to situations requiring flexibility. Students' nurturant qualities and commitment to care about people may be more and more difficult to express.

While the amount and character of academic work is the same for men and women, other aspects of the medical school experience are not necessarily the same. The social environment is often perceived differently by male and female students. For example, students learn how to function, in part, by identifying with people who act as models, particularly those who are seen as successful.[18] These include teachers, peers, those who care for patients, as well as patients themselves.[13,14,19-23] Since most medical school faculty members are still predominantly men, the male student can identify with other physicians and maintain a consistency with his own masculine identification. This is not true for the female student. She may have difficulty finding a woman physician who can be a role model, since there may not have been any in her past experience, nor are there many women faculty available in medical school at this time.[22,24-30] The number of women faculty remains low, particularly in the highest ranks. Current trends in academic appointments suggest that this will not change as rapidly in the near future as might be expected from the dramatic increase in women medical students and graduates.[31]

There are other differences in the experience of men and women. Women students have felt excluded, isolated,[22,32] and not regarded as serious.[22,33-35] While the changing peer culture of medical school may alter this picture, those women who are in training and practice continue to describe some absence of peer support and negative attitudes toward female physicians. Many women in medical training today continue to feel the subtle effects of institutional practices which were set up without them in mind.

The training years occur during that period of time when peers are freer to explore interpersonal relationships and commitments. Also impinging at this time are social and family pressures, and their own sex role expectations from past developmental experiences.[19,22,24,36-47] For women students and house officers this is particularly significant since the demands of training often seem, at that stage, to preclude intensive family involvement.[48] In the past, female physicians have chosen not to marry or have children, or they have limited their professional commitments.[5,30,34,35,37,49-51] Male students have not been constrained to make these choices.

Another set of differences in the experience for men and women derives from the implications and significance of choosing medicine as a career. For those who are choosing the unexpected or deviant pattern by going into medicine, the choice brings up conflict with many values which may seem to be external but also are internally maintained. Although there have been real cultural changes, with women receiving a great deal more support from their families than they did a decade ago, they still question what the experience will do to their "femininity," poorly defined and in flux as this concept may be.

There is a disparity between those traits which are considered traditionally "feminine" and those qualities considered important in the selection of students for medicine.[14,22,26,33,37,43,46,52] There is also a difference in the balance between nurturant wishes and achievement wishes for men and women in relation to medicine. Because medicine involves caretaking and nurturance, it allows for the expression of these needs in men while still reinforcing achievement needs and not compromising "masculine" goals. The situation is different for women. Although nurturant qualities have been considered traditionally "feminine," medicine in this country has been seen as an achievement-oriented, and therefore "masculine," field. Those women who have become physicians have found that conflicts concerning achievement and nurturance are of major importance.[42]

The assertiveness and independence which are supported and reinforced in men have been seen as less desirable in women. Medicine requires those qualities that are seen as traditionally "masculine," as well as "feminine" ones. Thus it is possible that women who have fit more traditional norms did not, in the past, consider medicine. As societal values change, however, a wider range of personality styles will be seen as acceptable and adaptive for both men and women. Those in medical training in the future will enter with different traits and values, perhaps making adaptation easier in some areas but more difficult in others, because of the rigidity of current training models. The motivation for the choice of medicine, and the supports available during the educational process, are important determinants of the capacity to adapt to its demands.[7,22,30,51,53,54] Thus while motivation appears to be high in both men and women, supports are not as readily available for women. This lack may contribute to a difference in the stress experienced.

PERSONALITY SIMILARITIES AND DIFFERENCES

Differences in personality, values, motivations, and attitudes between women and men have been examined for possible determinants of difference in their reactions. Unfortunately studies have largely looked at isolated variables or collections of "traits" and have not studied the nature of the experience in context, nor have they actually compared the stresses and the process of resolution in men and women. Studies do not entirely agree. For example, Cartwright[43-45] found differences between female medical students and the "traditional" norms for women in their emphasis on individuation, self-discovery, self-expression, and self-differentiation in work.

Freun et al.[46] also found differences, with male medical school applicants scoring higher on traits of "dominance," "exhibitionism," and "order," in the Personality Research Form they administered. Women had higher scores on "harm avoidance," "impulsivity," "nurturance," "understanding," and "need for change." Men and women applicants did not differ on aggression, autonomy, endurance, and affiliative traits, although these traits did separate men and women undergraduates.

McGrath and Zimet[55] have contradicted some of these findings. They found female students higher than males on self-confidence, autonomy, and aggression, while males rated themselves higher than did females on nurturance, affiliation, and deference. The authors speculate that the increased numbers of women and the effect of the women's movement, supporting increased assertiveness and untraditional career choices, account for their results. There is evidence that men and women medical students are more like each other in personality than they are like rejected medical school applicants and college students.[47] These trait studies, however, may not tell us a great deal about contemporary students or about the complex process of their development.

An important personality component which relates to the medical school experience concerns pressure toward achievement. Students who apply to medical school are generally high achievers and continue to be. As noted, there is evidence that this kind of achievement is viewed differently by men and women. Achievement and competition appear to be more conflicted issues for women. Women students internalize socially reinforced values concerning achievement and success and may project or externalize their conflicts about activity versus passivity. That is, they may feel that they cannot be active and aggressive, and they may attempt to suppress these traits. This in turn may affect their performances and choices, both in and outside of medical school.[22,39,56]

Horner[40,41] has defined the "motive to avoid success" as a manifestation of conflict between achievement orientation and traditional feminine goals. She reports that women who show a high "fear of success" perform more poorly in situations which are mixed sex, and in competitive achievement situations, than in noncompetitive but achievement-oriented situations. An important aspect of the conflict between achievement and "femininity" relates to the perceived cost of succeeding, in terms of human relationships.

DETERMINANTS OF SPECIALTY CHOICES

There have been few comparisons of specialty choice for men and women which follow students long enough to learn if a planned career path is the one actually chosen.

Women students struggle with their own interests and the realities of both being accepted and functioning well in training programs, as well as managing their careers in the future. Often the field of choice narrows by virtue of the desire of the female student not to be the person to achieve martyrdom by qualifying in a field which is particularly difficult for women.[22] Thus women often have not pursued their interest in surgical fields because the atmosphere of the institution training program is seen as hostile or unresponsive. They need to reconcile their interests in a field with the conditions of work in that field. Important concerns are the numbers of women in the field, the house, flexibility of time arrangement, and the specific ambience of the work.[5,26,33,35,37-39,42,48,49]

Even with some awareness of these, the real planning and the working out of future decisions such as marriage, pregnancy, child care, etc., are not usually confronted realistically until these events occur. At these stressful times, individuals and couples are likely to attempt to resolve the immediate crisis rather than to construct long-term strategies. The result may be detrimental both in terms of long-term career goals and family functioning. Even when people do plan, it is difficult to anticipate all eventualities.

In a dual-career family, a structure which fits most women in medicine, it is also often not possible for each partner to make plans and set individual goals, since these may not be consistent with the spouse's or family's needs. A traditional model generally holds in these families. The woman more often limits her aspirations to enable her spouse to fulfill his. This may limit the performance of women physicians. Several studies have indicated that among the factors correlating with professional performance in women, the number of children was inversely related to medical activity.[8,29,57]

Role proliferation and consequent role strain have been described in high-career woman.[58] This phenomenon has been repeatedly reported in women physicians. Heins et al.[59] have found that, despite the fact that the women physicians in the sample spent 90% as much time as men in medical work, they tended to assume full responsibility for home and family. The problems of integrating career and marriage have been considered by a number of authors,[28,32,33,60] all of whom have concluded that dual responsibilities result in role overload and conflict. Despite these problems, many women do not recognize the extent of their efforts nor do they find other solutions, and few report more than a year interruption in training or practice. While it is possible to conclude that there is no evidence that the stress is excessive,[3] from measurements of specific resulting pathology there is evidence of lower female achievement[29] in medicine.

A SURVEY OF HARVARD MEDICAL SCHOOL GRADUATES

A recent survey of current activities and concerns of Harvard Medical School graduates from 1967 to 1972, which included all the women and a matched sample of men, revealed that there were no major differences in marital status, number of children, or types of postgraduate training. The major areas of difference were that a larger number of women were working part-time, or in positions they viewed as compromises, based on family considerations.

It is of interest that 45% of the men, when answering a question about arrangements for the care of children, stated simply "wife" and another 10% reported that their wives had help. Obviously, this solution is not an available alternative for women physicians. Of the group of women, 65% had full-time household help and only one reported that her husband took primary responsibility. When asked about conflicts related to marital or family situation, women overwhelmingly reported their problems related to time pressures and desires to be with children, obtaining suitable jobs for both partners, and other dual-career issues. Another consideration mentioned by women was financial. They felt that the cost of obtaining good help was a serious problem, especially during the training period. Both men and women felt the need for more role models and counseling services of various kinds. Women were more specific in requests for contact with other women who had "done it" or for groups which could be both supportive and problem solving.[61]

While these data represent one group of physicians who are in the midst of a rapidly changing societal situation, it is important to note that they were all chosen for high achievement, leadership, and motivation, with a good history of adapting to serious challenges. Problems encountered might be even greater in less highly competitive and achieving students and physicians.

THERAPEUTIC APPROACHES

There are some potentially effective approaches which can alleviate existing problems, prevent future ones, and facilitate more optimal functioning of women and men as students and physicians. From our own survey of recent graduates, as well as from the literature, some possible directions suggest themselves.

Opportunities for discussion, counseling, and crisis intervention should be available to students and physicians. The young physicians in our study repeatedly cited the lack of such opportunities during medical school. Even though these are technically available to many, not every student finds ready access to faculty, advisors, counselors, therapists, or even peers.

Students and house officers would also benefit from access to practical information about the realities of medical practice, in a number of specialties. This would include discussion about how to set up a practice, as well as the specific problems and rewards which can be expected. Other areas which would benefit from concrete discussion and help with decision-making are those related to family considerations, e.g., child care.

For women, the availability of role models and the opportunity to exchange ideas and experiences appear to be extremely important. Although this is often repeated, it remains an unmet need. At the present time, when women enter practice they encounter fewer women than they did while they were in school. This is particularly true if they are in fields where there are few women, or if they move to relatively isolated areas.

In our experience, discussion groups have also been very useful not only in alleviating feelings of isolation, but also in facilitating the development of problem-solving skills. Medical student groups conducted by the authors have offered their members help with the stresses of separation from families, and in coping with painful past experiences. They have also focused on ways of handling the impact of clinical contact and the feelings evoked by patients.

Support groups, and possibly counseling, for spouses and families should be developed. These might help with marital strains. Creating opportunities where families could join house officers, such as at meals or evenings on call, if work pressure permits, would diminish the conflict for those women (and men) who juggle parenting responsibilities with medicine.

INSTITUTIONAL CHANGE

Change on an institutional level is needed to permit greater flexibility in training. Part-time programs, or more humane full-time programs will help all physicians, not only women. Training is a stressful and lonely experience, and depression may occur. Time demands exclude families and are cited as a reason for failures in marriages and close relationships.

In the clinical rotations and more consistently during the house officer period, the stress of work overload, fatigue, and lack of sleep is disruptive. Valko and Clayton[62] recently documented the relationship between lack of sleep and depression. The interns they studied felt less efficient in their work, "but more important were the feelings of help-lessness and actual incapacity they described." Friedman[63,64] has also correlated lack of sleep with decreased work efficiency. Counseling alone cannot change the stressful working conditions, but would help in anticipating the problems. An awareness that the experience is shared can be very supportive. In addition, some real changes in programs are indicated.

Decreasing the time demands of the house officer period has been seen as interfering with optimal training. Historically, this position has been stated and restated with every alteration in working and learning conditions. Students were admonished not to marry and they were told that changing from every other night on call to every third or fourth night would disrupt continuity of patient care. Each change has not been proven to be detrimental.

In the past, since there were few women in medicine, information on the relationship between medical training and childbearing was scant. Although most women physicians appear to postpone childbear-ing until after training, data on the particular problems, strains, and solutions have yet to be systematically examined. Our own data, based on a survey of Harvard and Tufts Medical School alumni, has indicated that women physicians do modify their career plans more often for family reasons than do their male counterparts. This group of alumni, however, grew up in a time when other societal changes had not taken place, so that there may be differences in the experiences of students currently in medical school.

Flexibility of programs and the recognition of the feelings and needs of trainees does not mean a diminished sense of responsiblity or readi-ness to serve and sacrifice time and effort when it is necessary. It would instead create a sense of respect for the physicians' emotional and physical well-being which would be reflected in the way they respect the feelings of patients.

PHYSICIANS AS PATIENTS

Physicians are generally reluctant to seek help early even when they are symptomatic. Among the major problems noted in treating "special" patients, including physicians, are the complexity of transference–countertransference problems. Changes in the authority relationships in medical practice might make it easier for physicians to seek help. If the physician could relinquish the omnipotent role, he or she perhaps would have fewer difficulties acknowledging problems. To the extent that the greater numbers of women entering medicine have an effect on the field, and possibly contribute to the development of a different image of the physician, the patterns of help-seeking of physicians may change and ultimately be beneficial to both physicians and patients.

CONCLUSION

As we look at the picture relating to women in medicine, several potential problem areas emerge. Despite the increasing numbers of women in the field, it remains male dominated, particularly in the academic hierarchy. Therefore those who teach medical students and are influential in their careers are likely to be men. The absence of role models and support for less traditional career directions is evident, and for some women may be distressing and limiting.

Time pressures and other demands make it necessary for women to postpone or find complex or difficult solutions to childbearing and childrearing, if they plan to combine this with training. Indications are that this causes modifications in their career plans more than for men. Further, most women in medicine who do have families experience considerable role strain. It is clear that institutional as well as personal solutions will be necessary in the future as women are increasingly involved in medical careers. As more women enter the field, stereotypes will change, including distribution in certain specialties. Presumably women and men will make more substantive contributions in a wide variety of fields.

REFERENCES

1. American Association of Medical Colleges Medical Student Information System, 1981.
2. Hugunin MB (ed): Helping the impaired physician, in *Proceedings of the AMA Conference on "The Impaired Physician: Answering the Challenge,"* Atlanta, Feb. 4–6, 1977.
3. Vincent M: Women physicians as psychiatric patients, *Can Psychiat Assoc J* 21:461–465, 1976.
4. Green RC, Caroll GJ, Buxton WD: *The Care and Management of the Sick and Incompetent Physician,* Springfield, Ill, Charles C Thomas, 1978.
5. Phelps C: Women in American medicine, *J Med Educ* 43:916–924, 1968.

6. Crowley AE (ed): Medical education in the U.S. *JAMA* 234:1338, 1975.
7. Adsett C: Psychological health of medical students in relation to the medical education process, *J Med Educ* 43:728–734, 1968.
8. Gove W, Tudor J: Adult sex roles and mental illness, *Am J Sociol* 78:812–835, 1973.
9. Weinberg E, Rooney J: Performance of female medical students. *J Med Educ* 48:240, 1973.
10. Steppacher RC, Mausner JS: Suicide in male and female physicians, *JAMA* 228:323–328, 1974.
11. Rosow I, Rose KD: Divorce among doctors, *J Marriage and Family* 34:587–598, 1972.
12. Berman E, Sacks S, Lief H: The two-professional marriage—a new conflict syndrome, *J Sex and Marriage Therapy* 1:242–253, 1975.
13. Lief H: Doctors and marriage: The special pressures, *Med World News* Feb. 7, 1977.
14. Kimball C: Medical education as a humanizing process, *J Med Educ* 48:71–77, 1973.
15. Lief HI, Young K, Spruiel V, et al: Psychodynamic study of medical students and their adaptational problems. *J Med Educ* 35: 696–704, 1960.
16. Nadelson C, Notman M: unpublished data.
17. Keniston K: The medical student, *Yale J Biol Med* 39:346–356, 1967.
18. Lucas CJ, Kelvin RP, Ojha AB: The psychological health of the pre-clinical medical student, *Br J Psychiat* 3:473–478, 1965.
19. McGuire FL: Psycho-social studies of medical students: A critical review, *J Med Educ* 41:424–445, 1961.
20. Miller GE: *Teaching and Learning in Medical School*, Cambridge, Mass, Harvard University Press, 1961.
21. Mudd JW, Siegel R: Sexuality—the experience and anxieties of medical students, *N Engl J Med* 281:1397–1404, 1967.
22. Notman M, Nadelson C: Medicine: A career conflict for women, *Am J Psychiat* 130:1123–1127, 1973.
23. Olmsted A: Products and by-products of a new community-based medical school. Unpublished manuscript, 1975.
24. Bowers J: Special problems of female medical students, *J Med Educ* 43:532–537, 1968.
25. Campbell M: *Why Would a Girl Go into Medicine?* New York, The Feminist Press, 1973.
26. Epstein, C: Encountering the male establishment: Sex-status limits on women's careers in the professions, *Am J Sociol* 15:6–9, 1975.
27. Hilberman E, Konanc J, Perez-Reyes M, et al: Support groups for women in medical school: A first-year program, *J Med Educ* 50:867–875, 1975.
28. Roeske N: The quest for role models by women medical students, *J Med Educ* 52:459–466, 1977.
29. Westling-Wikstrand H, Monk M, Thomas CB: Some Characteristics related to the career status of women physicians, *Johns Hopkins Med J* 127:273–286, 1970.
30. Williams P: Women in medicine: Some themes and variations. *J Med Educ* 46:584–591, 1971.
31. Witte M, Arem A, Hoquin M: Women physicians in the U.S. medical schools: A preliminary report, *JAMWA* 31:211–216, 1976.
32. Edwards M, Zimet C: Problems and concerns among medical students, 1975, *J Med Educ* 51:619–625, 1976.
33. Lopate C: *Women in Medicine*, Baltimore, Johns Hopkins Press, 1968, pp 27–35.
34. Matthew E: Attitude toward career and marriage, and development of life-style, *J Counsel Psychiat* 11:374–384, 1969.
35. Matthew MPH: Training and practice of women physicians, *J Med Educ* 45:1016–1024, 1970.

36. Cox, D: *Youth into Maturity.* New York, Mental Health Materials Center, 1970.
37. Cosa J, Coker RE Jr: The female physician in public health: Conflict and reconciliation of the sex and professional roles, *Social Soc Res* 49:294–305, 1965.
38. Nagley DL: Traditional and pioneer working mothers, *J Vocat Behav* 1:133, 1971.
39. Rosen-Hudson RA: Occupational role innovators and sex role attitudes, *J Med Educ* 49:554–561, 1974.
40. Horner M: Toward an understanding of achievement related conflicts in women, *J Soc Issues* 28:157–175, 1972.
41. Horner M: The motive to avoid success and the changing aspirations of college women, 1970, in Bardwick J (ed): *Readings on the Psychology of Women,* New York, Harper & Row, 1972, pp 62–67.
42. Notman M, Nadelson C, Bennett M: Achievement conflict in women: psychotherapeutic considerations, in Karger X (ed): *Proceedings of the 10th International Congress for Psychotherapy,* Basel, Switzerland, 1976.
43. Cartwright LK: Conscious factors entering into decisions of women to study medicine, *J Soc Issues* 282:201–215, 1972.
44. Cartwright LK: Personality differences in male and female medical students, *Psychiat in Med* 33:213–218, 1972.
45. Cartwright LK: The Personality and family background of a sample of women medical students at the, University of California. *J Am Med Wom Assoc* 27:260–261, 1972.
46. Fruen M, Rothman A, Steiner J: Comparison of characteristics of male and female medical school applicants, *J Med Educ* 49:137–145, 1974.
47. Roessler R, Collins MD, Forrest BS, et al: Sex similarities in successful medical school applicants, *JAMWA* 30:254–265, 1975.
48. Nadelson C, Notman M: Success and failure: Women as medical school applicants, *JAMWA* 29:167–172, 1974.
49. Rosenlund M, Oski F: Women in medicine, *Ann Intern* 66:1008–1012, 1967.
50. Shapiro C, Stilber B, Zelknoic A, et al: Careers of women physicians: A survey of women graduates from seven medical schools, 1945–1951, *J Med Educ* 43:1033–1040, 1968.
51. Cohen ED, Korper SP: Women in medicine: Exigencies in training career, *Connect Med* 40:103–110, 1976.
52. Duki WG: Study of medical school applicants, *J Med Educ* 46:837–857, 1971.
53. Hunter RCA, Schwartzman AE: A clinical view of study difficulties in a group of counselled medical students, *J Med Educ* 36:1295, 1961.
54. Sazlow G: Psychiatric problems of medical students, *J Med Educ* 31:27, 1956.
55. McGrath E, Zimet G: Sex differences in specialty attitudes and personality among medical students, and their implications. *Proceedings* of 15th Annual Conference of the AAMC on Research in Medical Education, San Francisco, Nov. 1976.
56. Nadelson C, Notman M: Success and failure: Women as medical school applicants, *JAMWA* 29:167–172, 1974.
57. Thomas CB: What becomes of medical students: The dark side, *Johns Hopkins Med J* 138:185–195, 1976.
58. Johnson F, Johnson C: Role strain in High commitment career women. *J Am Acad Psychoanalysis* 4(1):13-36, 1976.
59. Heins M, Smock M, Martindale L, Stein B, Jacobs J: A profile of the woman physician. *J Amer Med Assoc* 32(11):421-427, 1977.
60. Heins M, Smock S, Jacobs J, Stein M: Productivity of women physicians. *JAMA* 236:1961–1964, 1976.

61. Nadelson C, Notman M, Lowenstein P: The practice patterns, life styles, and stresses of women and men entering medicine: A follow-up study of Harvard Medical School graduates from 1967 to 1977. *J Am Med Wom Assoc* 34(11):400–406, 1979.
62. Valko R, Clayton P: Depression in internship. *Dis Nerv Syst* 36:26–29, 1975.
63. Friedman R, Kornfeld D, Bigger R: Psychological problems associated with sleep deprivation in interns. *J Med Ed* 48:436-441, 1973.
64. Friedman R, Bigger R, Kornfeld D: The intern and sleep loss. *N Engl J Med* 285:201–203, 1971.

3

Problems of Drug Addiction and Alcoholism among Physicians

THOMAS G. WEBSTER

Problems of addiction and alcoholism among physicians now merit the most concerted special action by physicians individually and collectively. Physicians are at much higher risk than the general population, particularly for narcotic and sedative addiction. Despite a relatively high incidence, the numbers involved are sufficiently small to warrant a concerted focus and action. Prevention, earlier intervention, and more effective rehabilitation are demonstrably feasible and await more intensive implementation.

Preventable secondary complications take an extremely heavy toll on the afflicted physicians, their families, and their patients. The total loss of resources to their communities and the cost to the public is large. In addition to reported cases of physician drug addiction and alcoholism, an estimated 15,000 undetected or unreported cases also exist among physicians in the United States. Based on available studies, and if earlier estimates are unmodified, 1 of 10 physicians will become dependent on psychoactive drugs or alcohol sufficient to impair the practice of medicine at some time during their careers. One of 100 physicians will become narcotic addicts at some time during their careers, and 1 of 10 physician addicts or alcoholics will commit suicide.[1] To measure this in terms of cost, it would require one medical school graduating class of 100 graduates and all of its living alumni at a training cost of $8 million per year to replace the unfulfilled functions of the addicted and alcoholic physicians.

Substance abuse and addiction physiologically and psychologically erode the physician's voluntary control and accentuate the importance of

THOMAS G. WEBSTER ● Department of Psychiatry and Behavioral Sciences, and Department of Child Health and Development, George Washington University School of Medicine and Health Sciences, Washington, D.C.

external influences by colleagues and family. More concerted attention by private psychiatrists and organized medicine is strongly indicated in the best traditions of humane care, early intervention, and public responsibility. The demonstration of reduced incidence and severity of complications has already occurred in some states. Accountability of psychiatrists, other physicians, and American medicine now has high visibility in Congress, in the health industry, and in public. The feasible and demonstrable results of more intensive concerted action would be especially timely.

INCIDENCE AND PREVALENCE*

The incidence of narcotic addiction in physicians has been estimated to be 30–100 times greater than in the general population.[2,3] Alcoholism among physicians is less reliably reported but is believed similar to that of the general population of comparable age, sex, and socioeconomic status, and the incidence exceeds that of drug addiction. Physicians are not so different in their rate of alcoholism compared to the general population as they are different in their rate of narcotic addiction.[4] About one-half of physician alcoholics develop other drug dependencies.[5]

As emphasized above, approximately 1 physician out of 100 becomes a narcotic addict at some time during his or her career.[6,7] Roughly 7% of physicians are or will become alcoholics at some time during their careers.[4] In private psychiatric settings, such as the Menninger Clinic, the Mayo Clinic, and the Homewood Sanitarium in Ontario, approximately one-half of the physicians admitted were dependent on alcohol or drugs, and one-third of physician outpatients were dependent on alcohol or drugs.[3,8,9] The median age of onset is about 43 (median range 36–46 years in different studies).[2,3] Addicted physicians have been in practice an average of 18 years at the time of discovery of addiction.[2] The most common narcotic abused by physicians is meperidine (Demerol), though morphine was more common in earlier years and newer drugs are now becoming more common.[2,10] The most common medical specialties in most reports are general practitioners and internists with a comparably high number of surgeons in the Mayo and Homewood

---

* Statistical data and trends are reasonably consistent and reliable for the points emphasized in this chapter. However, many limitations exist in comparability, reliability, and projections of available data, which come from many different years and settings. The limitations in comparing data are best illustrated in the statistics of physician suicides by different medical specialties.

reports.[2,8,9] No single specialty is strongly disproportionately represented nationwide (see footnote, page 32).

COURSE OF ILLNESS AND TREATMENT: ASSOCIATED FACTORS

Many associated factors complicate the onset and course of drug addiction and alcoholism of physicians. These complications greatly add to the morbidity and mortality and to the cost for all concerned, but they also provide guides for earlier intervention and more effective treatment.

In the study by Green et al. of 46 cases of drug addiction in the state of Virginia, physical pain and illness, usually chronic, was the main precipitating factor in 22 cases.[2] Less common factors included family tragedy (such as death of wife or child), an addicted spouse, or situational stress such as overwork and marital problems. Modlin and Montes made a helpful distinction in reporting separately on the physician addicts' views of factors in the onset and the authors' psychiatric views of the onset of addiction.[3] Other authors have questioned the common tendency for physicians to view "overwork" as a major precipitating factor. A study by Putnam and Ellinwood of the Lexington PHS Hospital found that physician addicts changed location twice as frequently as a control group of physicians. The change of location accentuates the common problem of isolation of the physician and family.[10]

Evidence of childhood, family, and personality problems, antedating admission to medical school and predisposing to adjustment problems as physicians, and later to substance abuse and addictions, has been reported in several studies. Modlin and Montes report such findings on the basis of psychoanalytic and psychodynamic perspectives of their cases.[3] Other authors report similar historical and psychiatric diagnostic findings. Post hoc findings of psychopathologic predispositions, however valid, are always subject to some question as to specificity and relevance for addiction. All authors have also pointed out the special overdeterminants for physician drug abuse compared to the general population. Several authors have indicated the differences between physicians and other addicts in terms of lesser degrees of predisposing psychopathology and greater work-related and situational determinants in physician cases. A related point is the relatively good prognosis for physician addicts and alcoholics, given adequate and timely treatment, as compared to dim and stereotyped views commonly held about narcotic addiction and alcoholism. However, depression and immature or disturbed personality traits are commonly associated with addiction and

alcoholism among physicians. Psychotherapy and supportive relationships at home and work are found very important while interrupting the
drug and alcohol dependency.

The reports by Vaillant et al. of longitudinal studies with controls
are of special relevance to the above issues. In their first study they
found that over a 20-year period a group of 45 physicians did indeed
"take more tranquilizers, sedatives and stimulants than 90 matched
[nonphysician] controls," though the physicians "drank alcoholic bev-
erages and smoked cigarettes to the same extent as the controls." All
subjects had been selected for study as college sophomores "because of
better than average physical and psychological health."[11]

Using the same population base, the second study found that 47
physicians,

> especially those involved in patient care, were more likely than controls [79
> nonphysicians, matched socioeconomically with the physicians] to have rela-
> tively poor marriages, to use drugs and alcohol heavily, and to obtain psy-
> chotherapy. Although these difficulties are often assumed to be occupational
> hazards of medicine, their presence or absence appeared to be strongly
> associated with life adjustment before medical school. Only the physicians
> with the least stable childhoods and adolescent adjustments appeared vul-
> nerable to these occupational hazards.[6]

However, the sample included only four physicians and one control
subject in which the drug or alcohol abuse was reportedly severe
enough to interfere with employment of family relations. Unlike many
other studies, this study was not conducted on an inpatient service.
Apparently the psychopathology of these physicians was much less
serious, or the emotional supports much more effective, compared to
the physicians with narcotic addiction and alcoholism described in other
studies above. However, this follow-up study of "healthy students"
reinforces the strong indications for earlier intervention and for predictive studies of high-risk students and controls.

Associated psychiatric diagnoses in reported studies of physician
addiction and alcoholism most commonly include neuroses, personality
disorders, and depression, and less commonly schizophrenia and
organic brain syndrome. Reported incidences of the different associated
diagnoses vary according to the type of addictive group being studied,
i.e., whether the group subjects are primarily sedative and/or narcotic
addicts, alcoholics, dependents on other drugs, or some other combination. Reported associated diagnoses are naturally fewer in studies where
drug addiction and alcoholism are used as singular diagnoses. For example, in such studies "personality disorders" were relatively rare, such as

5%–10%. One example where all cases had an associated psychiatric diagnosis is the Virginia study of 43 narcotic addicts: neuroses and personality disorders, 24 cases; depression, 11; manic-depressive, 2; and other psychoses, 9.[2]

A follow-up of New York state narcotic addicts, not just physicians, reported 35%–42% on stable abstinence after 20 years; 23% had died. Among physician suicides, Blachly et al. reported "heavy drinking" or "alcoholic" associated with 39% of cases, and 19% were drinking at the time of death. "Drug dependence or severe abuse was a factor in 19%, and only 33% were said not to have used drugs." About 10% of U.S. physician addicts commit suicide.[12] In the Virginia study 27 physician addicts had returned to private practice, 6 remained in institutional work, and 11 had their licenses revoked due to repeated relapse.

The outlook for physician addicts is notably improved by systematic and individualized attention which provides confidentiality, active treatment, and external controls if necessary. The earlier and more confidentially such attention can be established on a voluntary basis, the better. Obviously this is easier said than done, but more can be done on a private basis. Awareness and assurance that effective confidential treatment is available can make a difference. As backup, newer and more active peer review, ethics committees and similar medical committees, state licensure boards, and hospitals have been taking a stance toward more therapeutic interventions. At more advanced stages of physician narcotic addiction, rehabilitation rates have been reported best when there is compulsory follow-up as well as active treatment. Reports from the California State Board of Medical Examiners and Virginia recommend that compulsory follow-up is best handled at the state board level, which includes removal or restricting licensure, continued enforceable surveillance and reevaluation, mandatory removal of narcotic license, as well as treatment and continuing education.[2,7] Under these conditions, rehabilitation rates improved from 27%–28% in earlier studies to 72% successful rehabilitation in Virginia and 92% successful rehabilitation in California.

EARLY INTERVENTION

A major problem is the lack of earlier detection and treatment in spite of the known high risk for drug addiction and alcoholism among physicians. Early problems may be manifest in medical school or residency training. The more serious cases, which are the source of most clinical reports and statistics, appear in more advanced stages of physicians' careers. In reported studies, only about one-third of physician narcotic addicts are reported within 1 year of onset. Known factors which increase addiction rates among physicians include: (1) easier access to drugs; (2) familiarity with clinical use of drugs and with many patients' experiences; (3) professional and family life stresses; (4) psychological factors in individual physicians; and (5) concealment and avoidance factors by which physicians are reluctant to report themselves or colleagues in early stages.

Waring reported:

> The case records of 30 physicians and 30 nurses hospitalized for emotional illness were compared with a control group of psychiatric inpatients matched for age, sex, and admission diagnosis. Drug abuse and depression were found more frequently in the doctor–nurse group although the difference was not statistically significant for depression. Family history of psychiatric illness, disturbed childhood, and past history of psychiatric treatment were the major predisposing factors to illness in the doctor–nurse group, and professional role was seldom the contributing or precipitating factor. Physicians and nurses were significantly more likely to have attempted suicide and abused drugs before admission and were more often admitted informally, from out-of-town, and their families were seldom involved in the treatment process. These findings suggest that being a "special patient" acts as a perpetuating factor contributing to problems in treatment.[13]

Bissell and Jones* reported on

> interviews with 98 recovered alcoholic physicians, all of whom had been entirely abstinent for a minimum of one calendar year. Psychiatry was the only specialty clearly overrepresented. [Percentage of each specialty in the sample of recovered alcoholic physicians was compared to percentage of all U.S. physicians in that specialty: general practice, 24.5%/22%; internal medicine, 13.3%/14%; surgery, 9.2%/10%; psychiatry, 17.4%/6%; obstetrics-gynecology, 9.2%/6%; etc.*] A disproportionate number of subjects reported high standing in their medical school classes. Nearly half of the sample had experienced difficulty with drugs other than alcohol. While legal sanctions and admission to health care and correctional institutions were common among this group, relatively little formal response of a disciplinary nature from colleagues or medical organizations was reported.[4]

---

* This is the only U.S. study among those reviewed be present author in which "psychiatry overrepresentation" was found among physicians with drug addiction and alcoholism. From different studies in different settings, no consistent or reliable overall trend is reported, or appears significant nationwide. Ophthalmologists, anesthesiologists, psychiatrists, surgeons, and internists have been "overrepresented" in different individual reports.

Additionally, 49% of the subjects had been arrested, 37.8% had been jailed, and 19.4% had lost their driver's license. These physicians accumulated a total of 219 arrests and 170 jailings.[4]

An additional factor in problems of physician addiction and early intervention is physicians' use of sedatives, minor tranquilizers, and stimulants. Vaillant et al. reported that 62% of doctors, compared to 32% of controls, used such medications moderately, such as daily use of tranquilizers for less than 1 month[11]; 11% of doctors, compared to 29% of controls, reported no use of such medications. For comparison, physicians were the same as controls in rates of smoking and use of alcohol in moderation. Some of these differences presumably represent the physician functioning as an educated consumer, not necessarily detrimentally, rather than as abuser of medications. A helpful distinction would be those physicians who use drugs in moderation "successfully" compared to those prone to addiction. A likely hypothesis would be that those who pay insufficient attention to their emotional needs are more prone to addiction.

The Georgia Disabled Doctors Program of earlier intervention presents an attractive alternative to the above two examples of "special patient," relative neglect by colleagues, and police intervention. It also appears to be a preferable alternative to the more compulsory approach in California and Virginia, though state boards must intervene with compulsory measures as a last resort. Dudley and Talbott reported that the new Georgia plan has had a

> 100% success rate in helping the chemically dependent physician in treatment and adjustment. . . . in the first 2 years, 20 sick doctors throughout Georgia had been found who voluntarily suspended practicing medicine, successfully went through treatment and came back to active work, without one name being revealed to the state licensing board. The success of the Georgia plan has been widely publicized throughout the state, thus case finding is becoming easier.[15]

The Georgia State Medical Association allocates a substantial portion of its budget to support of this program. Talbott, the program chairman, is also the founder of the Caduceus Club in Georgia for physicians recovering from chemical dependencies. Members and families meet once a week at various locales to provide moral support and help with reentry into practice. Recovering alcoholics are encouraged to attend Alcoholics Anonymous as well as Caduceus Club meetings. The program is young, and not every physician, state, or region would necessarily find this approach the answer. However, the principles of early intervention, colleague support, "voluntary" participation, family involvement, and follow-up contacts, combined with treatment and assistance in work rehabilitation, are sound.

RECOMMENDATIONS

1. Medical school admissions committees may select out applicants who have predicted high risk for drug addiction, alcoholism, and other psychiatric problems. Such action has been proposed by those concerned with decreasing the number of physician addicts. Selection processes already accomplish this to some degree with more extreme risk applicants. More predictive and longitudinal studies are indicated for a variety of purposes. Retrospective assessment of known addicts and alcoholics is not the same as prediction and does not have comparable control cases for students with similar risk at the time of admission but who did not become such casualties. Unless or until better predictors of noncognitive, behavioral, and emotional factors in career performance are available, the present state of the art of selection is not sufficiently specific. A two-edged hazard exists. Greater stringency on "mental health" grounds might well accentuate an inappropriate bias of admissions committees. However, predictive pilot projects, with experimental and control groups, should be conducted on a longitudinal study basis. The Vaillant et al. study is relevant, but for a *low*-risk selection of students.[6]

2. More intensive educational efforts can and should be made in medical schools, residency training, and continuing education of physicians. The educational objectives should include both knowledge and attitude change. Knowledge would be in the nature of information described in this chapter and related references. Attitude change requires additional educational methods, involving affective, interpersonal, and experiential learning, usually in small groups with peers, expertly led. Current examples occur in areas such as human sexuality and death and dying. The attitudinal objectives should focus on: (1) high-risk signs and feelings involving self-awareness and greater readiness to ask for help when indicated; and (2) altered values and sensitivity in recognizing and dealing more appropriately with colleagues and peers who may be avoiding seeking help when indicated. A matter-of-fact attitude is desired, erring neither in glossing and avoidance nor in moralizing or an oversolicitous therapeutic zeal. When dealing with students or physicians already manifesting substance-abuse symptoms, a premium should be placed on genuine personal and professional respect, for some degree of embarrassment and humiliation is inevita-

ble. Training materials and methods should be developed and demonstrated on a trial pilot basis with evaluation, preferably by experts such as psychiatric educators and their colleagues. Successful materials and methods should be prepared, and teacher training made available, for broader distribution to medical schools and other training programs for physicians.

3. Earlier case finding and intervention at medical student and residency levels should be pursued. Such activity would also better prepare their peer colleagues for early intervention during their later careers. One example: Knott recently initiated the "Impaired Student Plan" in cooperation with the University of Tennessee administration.[16] The plan is university wide, but the majority of cases have come from the medical school. Courses have been initiated on alcohol and drug dependence for students. The Faculty–Student Council has encouraged the concept "you are your brother's keeper" to help find the impaired student. Treatment resources outside the university are used instead of the Student Health Service in order to assure greater confidentiality.

4. Practicing psychiatrists should be more available and collaborate with medical colleagues. Psychiatrists should develop expertise in treating physician-patients. Effective approaches to problems of confidentiality, family involvement, and acceptable external controls at earlier stages of drug dependence and alcoholism would be part of the expertise. Habituated reliance by physician-patients on self-medication with psychoactive drugs or "moderation" alcohol should be firmly dealt with as the double jeopardy it is, whatever the associated psychodynamic factors. Several reports based on experiences of physician addicts and alcoholics indicate that psychiatrists did not see the patient's earlier drug or alcohol abuse as "the problem," and hence failed to interrupt that problem while attending to other aspects of the patient's problems. Therapeutic alliance with the physician-patient's own capacity for self-awareness and acceptance of at least partial need for external controls (via psychiatrist, other treating physicians, family, or trusted colleagues) should receive special attention. Beyond a certain point the therapist function should be separated from the external control functions, which can be carried by other medical colleagues. Contingencies should be faced openly with the physician-patient in a matter-of-fact manner. That is, the contingency should be made explicit as to what action the treating physician will take if the physician-patient appears to be becoming more victimized by his or her own self-defeating behavior while in treatment.

Naturally, the essence of best treatment is based on a maximum of trust and a minimum of threat. Genuine personal and professional respect is crucial. Cultivation of an effective alliance with the healthier self-preservative aspects of the patient's ego functions is also crucial. Difficult therapeutic dilemmas are involved. Experienced psychiatrists should be publishing more on psychotherapeutic and treatment-management experience and guidelines specifically addressed to problems of drug abuse and alcoholism of physicians.

5. Since many patients are already receiving successful treatment at all stages, from minor abuse of drugs and alcohol to advanced addiction and alcoholism, physicians and other health workers should have access as patients to "treatment as usual." "Special" consideration should involve the same elements of privacy, confidentiality, trust, and sensitivity—combined with external controls when indicated—as with any other patient, with due regard that some physicians and patients are more vulnerable to public interest or occupational exposure than others.

6. Prevention and treatment measures for practicing physicians should aim at earlier detection, with publication of the signs in medical literature, and earlier intervention. Earlier intervention should more commonly include work with physicians' spouses and families, with allied work colleagues in some settings, and consultation/education to medical group practices and institutional settings where physicians work.

7. Psychiatric educators, administrators, organization officials, and peer review committees should be mobilized to take more initiative and concerted action pertaining to problems of drug abuse and alcoholism among psychiatrists. Psychiatrists should also be more active in organized efforts of medical schools, other specialty societies, and general medical organizations. All psychiatrists should make it a point to talk informally with friends and colleagues about known problems among acquaintances—*not gossip* but respectful, confidential thought about tactful inquiries and approaches and by whom with whom.

8. District branches of the American Psychiatric Association and their medical counterparts should undertake more studied and intensive initiatives in education, treatment, and organized professional responsibility pertaining to all stages of physician drug and alcohol abuse. Legal counsel may be indicated for some issues. The AMA and state medical societies, such as in New York and other states already mentioned, are sponsoring activities to bring more thoughtful and concerted action, including model legislation.[17-21]

9. The American Psychiatric Association, American Medical Association, and similar national medical organizations should continue and augment their efforts with targeted measurable objectives. For example, a current base of data at local, state, or national level should be made available. Targeted objectives would be to increase the useful data avail-

able, with due regard for confidentiality, plus demonstrable decline in narcotic addiction, alcoholism, and perhaps associated suicides among physicians. An initial rise in reported incidence via better case finding and reporting should be anticipated. Pilot projects, demonstrations, and evaluations should be undertaken at the national and state level. I would hope that some such projects would build upon and utilize grant-supported projects of appropriate alcoholic, drug abuse, and mental health administration branches, state agencies, and private foundations, as well as funds from the relevant societies.

By 1982, recommended types of action are occurring nationwide.[22-27] Although this is encouraging, much remains to be done, and continuity of effort is crucial—beyond the recent flush of "discovery" of the impaired physician.

SUMMARY

In summary, the high risk of drug abuse and alcoholism among physicians is now well documented and receiving wider attention, more effective treatment, and organized professional self-control. Many additional measures for more effective prevention and earlier intervention, treatment, and rehabilitation are available. Psychiatrists have a crucial role in treatment, education, and consultation. More intensive educational, therapeutic, and organizational efforts should receive concerted attention by psychiatrists and their colleagues. Relevant studies, illustrations, and recommendations are described. Targeted baseline data and program objectives should be implemented for reducing the incidence and prevalence of the more visible and serious cases. This would have the valuable side-effect of bringing attention to earlier intervention, preventive education, and attitude change at all levels of medical education and practice. Other victims of drug abuse and alcoholism would benefit by a change in the more traditional physician attitudes and the mobilized treatment resources. The self-accountability and image of psychiatrists, other physicians, and American medicine would be enhanced.

REFERENCES

1. Palmer, RE: The impaired physician: Answering a challenge. President's introduction, AMA Department of Mental Health / Medical Association of Georgia Conference, Atlanta, Feb. 1977.
2. Green RC, Carroll GJ, Buxton WD: Drug addiction among physicians: The Virginia experience. JAMA 236:1372–1375, 1976.

3. Modlin HC, Montes A: Narcotics addiction in physicians. *Am J Psychiat* 121:358–363, 1964.
4. Bissell L, Jones, RW: The alcoholic physician: A survey. *Am J Psychiat* 133:1142–1146, 1976.
5. Vincent MO (cited in): Mental illness: Special risk. *Med World News* April 25, 1969, pp 42–44.
6. Vaillant GE, Sobowale NC, McArthur C: Some psychologic vulnerabilities of physicians. *N Engl J Med* 287:372–375, 1972.
7. Jones LE, Thompson W: How 92% beat the dope habit. *Bull Los Angeles Co Med Assoc* 88:19–40, 1958.
8. Duffy, JC, Litin EM: Psychiatric morbidity of physicians. *JAMA* 189:989–992, 1964.
9. Vincent MO, Robinson EA, Latt L: Physicians as patients: Private psychiatric hospital experience. *Can Med Assoc J* 100:403–412, 1969.
10. Putnam PL, Ellinwood EH Jr: Narcotic addiction among physicians: A ten year follow-up. *Am J Psychiat* 122:745–748, 1966.
11. Vaillant GE, Brighton JR, McArthur C: Physicians' use of mood-altering drugs: a 2-year follow-up report. *N Engl J Med* 282:365–372, 1970.
12. Blachly PH, Disher W, Roduner G: Suicide by physicians. *Bull Suicidology, December 1968*, pp 1–18.
13. Waring EM: Medical professionals with emotional illness. *Psychiat J Univ Ottawa* 2:161–164, 1977.
14. Dudley JC, Talbott GD: Disabled doctors program. Paper presented at conference in Atlanta, 1977.
15. Talbott, GD: The disabled doctors program of Georgia. *Alc: Clin Exp Res* 1:143–146, 1977.
16. Knott, DH: Medical students: Opportunities for prevention. Paper presented to AMA conference, Atlanta, Feb. 1977.
17. AMA Council on Mental Health: The sick physician. *JAMA* 223:684–687, 1973.
18. Medical Society of the State of New York Physicians' Committee: Special report: Proposed plans, noncoercive and coercive approaches. *N Y State J Med* Feb. 1975, pp 420–423.
19. Gitlow SE: The disabled physician—his care in New York State. *Alc: Clin and Exp Res* 1:131–134, 1977.
20. Newsom JA: Help for the alcoholic physician in California. *Alc: Clin and Exp Res* 1:135–137, 1977.
21. Johnston GP: The impaired physician: A treatment problem. *J. of Ind State Med Assoc* 71:1058–1060, 1978.
22. Johnson RP, Connelly JC: Addicted physicians: A closer look. *JAMA* 245:253–257, 1981.
23. Tokarz, JP, Bremer W, Peters K *et al.: Beyond survival.* Resident Physician Section of the AMA, Chicago, 1979.
24. Report of the Fourth National Conference on the Impaired Physician. *AMA Impaired Physician Newsletter.* January, 1981:1.
25. Spickard A, Billings FT: Alcoholism in a medical-school faculty. *N Engl J Med* 305:1646–1648, 1981.
26. Herrington RE, Benzer DC, Jacobson GR *et al.:* Treating substance-use disorders among physicians. *JAMA* 247:2253–2257, 1982.
27. Smith RJ, Steindler MS: The psychiatrist's role with the impaired physician. *Psychiatric Journal of the University of Ottawa* 7:3-7, 1982.

4

Physician Suicide
The Psychiatrist's Role

DAVID W. PREVEN

Suicide, a tragic consequence of physician impairment, looms in its seriousness because of its finality. In addition to the personal loss, it denies society of the contributions of one of its highly trained and needed members. Disturbing to lay persons and professionals alike is the realization that physicians, revered as caretakers of others, can care so little for themselves. This chapter contains a description of the scope of physician suicide, an outline of some of the special problems which are pertinent and some suggestions for management.

SCOPE OF THE PROBLEM

Since a 1964 editorial in the *British Medical Journal*,[1] the topic of physician suicide has been the subject of numerous articles both here and abroad.[2-7] A careful review of these and previous papers[8-12] leads to the conclusion that statistics purporting to show a high rate of physician suicide are *unfounded*, on the basis of recent evidence. Three recent critical overviews of physician suicide[13-15] all conclude that the statistical analysis in many of the papers is inadequate and misleading. Deficiences in the methodology include small samples, brief time period of data collection, inadequate controls for age and sex, and insufficient standardization of criteria for sample and reference groups.

For the present, three separate questions emerge from a review of the literature on physician suicide. First, are the rates of suicide for male physicians different from those for nonphysician controls? Second, how do the rates for women physicians compare to those for other women

DAVID W. PREVEN ● Department of Psychiatry, Albert Einstein College of Medicine of Yeshiva University, Bronx, New York.

and for male physicians? Finally, are suicide rates in some medical specialties, especially psychiatry, higher than in others?

The first question, concerning suicide in male physicians compared to other men, is the easiest to answer. A recent study by Rich and Pitts[16] confirms the findings from several previous reports that there is no difference between the suicide rate for male physicians and age-matched men in the U.S. Their study, national in scope, examined 544 suicides over 5 years, 1967–1972. Their rate of 35.7 suicides per 100,000 male physicians does not differ from that in same period for the general population of white men over 25, i.e., 34.6 per 100,000. They add that the most frequent method of suicide, poisoning, is consistently reported in all studies. Only the study by Rose and Rosow[17] in 1973 suggested that the rate for doctors was appreciably higher. In contrast to the Rich and Pitts work, Rose and Rosow's report was limited to a 3-year study period in California and included 48 suicides.

The second question, about the rate of suicide for female physicians, has generated more controversy. The issue is not whether female physicians have a higher suicide rate than nonphysician women. Three studies[18-20] confirm that the suicide rate for women doctors is 3–4 times that of nonphysician peers. Moreover, there is agreement that the rate for female physicians is similar to the rate for male physicians. Controversy has resulted from the statement by Pitts et al.[20] that 65% of woman physicians have an affective disorder. They arrived at this conclusion by linking some unreplicated reports suggesting, first, that all suicides were the result of primary affective disorders,[21] and second, that 10% of female affective disorders ended in suicide.[22] The 65% figure resulted from dividing 6.5 (percent of woman physician's deaths attributed to suicide), by 10 (the proportion of death attributed to suicide among women diagnosed as having a primary affective disorder). This publication stimulated a barrage of letters critizing their assumptions and methodology.[23] Whatever the reasons for the elevated suicide rate in women physicians, the finding is established; it is also observed among other women professionals.[24] These observations refer to suicide mortality (fatal acts). Little is known about the suicide morbidity (attempts) of female physicians. This is important because in the general population women attempt suicide more often than do men, but their attempts are less often fatal. Men, with fewer suicide attempts, still kill themselves more often than do women.

Certainly the experience of being a woman in medicine has changed markedly in the last 10 years. The previous male-to-female class ratio of 10 to 1 is now closer to 3 or 4 to 1. A peer group now exists which can provide formal and informal support during the arduous training experience.

Finally, there is the third question about physician suicide; whether there are higher rates for certain specialties. Craig and Pitts in 1968[25] suggested that psychiatrists had a higher suicide rate than did physicians in other specialties. However, the numbers were too small to demonstrate significance. Subsequent reports emphasized the statistical problems and failed to confirm that psychiatrists or psychiatric residents had a higher suicide rate. A recent study by Rich and Pitts is the first in which the numbers are large enough to observe statistical significance; they reviewed 18,730 consecutive physician deaths from 1967 to 1972.[26] According to their report, board-certified psychiatrists killed themselves at twice the expected rate. When "physicians with a preference for the practice of psychiatry" were observed, the same trend was found. Although statistically significant, this difference was not as great as for board-certified psychiatrists. No other group of board-certified specialists demonstrated higher-than-expected suicide rates. To account for the increased rates among psychiatrists, they hypothesized that physicians with a primary affective disorder tend to select psychiatry in preference to other fields.

The current evidence concerning physician suicide may be summarized as follows:

1. Suicide occurs in male physicians at the same rate as for age-matched controls in the United States.
2. Female physicians have a suicide rate 3–4 times that of nonphysician women but a rate similar to male physicians.
3. Psychiatrists appear to be overrepresented in the percentage of physician deaths due to suicide.

PROBLEMS IN MANAGEMENT OF THE SUICIDAL PHYSICIAN

Regardless of the statistical uncertainties of physician suicide, psychiatrists must contend with the weighty issue of its management. Suicidal behavior, in general, is one of the most challenging clinical problems for psychiatrists. When a medical colleague becomes suicidal, the issues become more complex and difficult. The doctor is a special patient; that special status influences each phase of management.

A crucial first step in salvaging the suicidal doctor is identifying the distressed individual, as the following clinical vignette illustrates:

> An esteemed internist in his 40's, married, with children, was found dead from a drug overdose in a motel a short distance from his home. Neither family, colleagues or patients suspected the inner turmoil that resulted in this man's killing himself.

The identification of the doctor in emotional distress is often delayed or missed altogether. Both lay persons and professionals resist recognizing that caretakers in the community can themselves be in need of care. For doctors it may mean abandoning a comforting if erroneous notion that the role of physician provides protection from illness. Character traits that contribute to success in medicine—self-reliance, perseverance, self-sacrifice, and, perhaps, suppression of feelings—become risk factors when the physician faces emotional difficulty. Patients, colleagues, and even family can regard the doctor as almost omnipotent. When an individual is surrounded by such expectations, it is difficult to acknowledge inner turmoil and ask for help. The doctor may maintain a calm facade while hopelessness grows, unchecked by contact with another whose perspective is not distorted by depressive feelings. Subtle pleas for help may go unnoticed because those around the troubled doctor cannot imagine the degree of inner strife in one perceived as so strong. The most important consideration in identifying the potential suicide is accepting that anyone, even an esteemed colleague, can be vulnerable to suicidal intention.[27] The development of this capacity in doctors is a key step toward earlier identification of a colleague in trouble. Premonitory signs may appear as a change in work habits and efficiency or subtle differences in temperament. The physician prepared to explore such clues tactfully may avert a tragic outcome.

One strategy for early identification is to encourage the physician to seek help. This approach should begin in medical school. As part of their career preparation, students should be informed about the emotional demands of a physician's work and the signs and symptoms that suggest personal difficulties.

A recent survey of the incidence of suicide in American medical students showed statistical patterns similar to those characterizing graduate physicians.[28] Male medical students had a suicide rate similar to a non-student age-matched sample. The suicide rate of female medical students was similar to that of their male colleagues and 2–3 times greater than that of the non-student women of similar age. Identifying the middle of the sophomore year as a time of particular stress, these authors suggested implementing educational and preventive programs on depression and suicide then. Medical students are notably resistant to seeking help; one goal of such programs should be to improve that situation. Students need to be able to recognize the special stresses on marital and family relationships that a medical career can produce.

Woman professionals may experience severe career pressures as they anticipate or attempt to manage the roles of spouse, mother, and

doctor. During medical school, support groups that provide an opportunity to share problems and possible solutions should be readily available. Training programs should encourage future physicians to regard
asking for needed help as positive and a sign of strength. Given the
number of people who will rely on the doctor, it is a professional's
responsibility to develop this self-awareness.

Whether the troubled doctor is self-referred or identified by a colleague, effective intervention remains challenging, as the following vignette illustrates.

> Two doctors, brothers, were found dead in their apartment, finally ending a
> prolonged downhill course of drug abuse. The press castigated the staff of
> the prestigious eastern hospital in which the physicians had practiced for not
> acting sooner in curtailing the doctors' work when it became apparent that
> there had been many early signs of impaired performance. There was also
> outrage that two doctors, identified by colleagues as being seriously ill, could
> slip through the health care system to their death.

Certainly, if intervention is to succeed at all, it should occur early
before self-esteem, personal relationships, and professional resources
have been devastated. Yet it is difficult to approach a colleague whom
one suspects of being in serious emotional distress. There are risks.
What if the physician angrily rejects the expression of concern? What
will be the consequences of another perceived assault on a faltering
sense of self-esteem? Could a poorly handled confrontation precipitate a
suicide? These are chances that must be taken, however, because inaction can result in tragic consequences as well.

The question of who should approach the doctor is a sensitive one.
While a colleague who is also a friend would be ideal, the series of events
leading to the desperate state usually has been preceded by withdrawal
from friends and often family as well. For such cases an older, respected
member of the medical community may prove the appropriate person to
approach the doctor.[29] This crucial initial contact requires a careful blend of
understanding, tact, and firmness. At this point the issues of confidentiality
and responsibilities emerge. Especially when the doctor's disturbed pattern
includes alcohol or drug abuse, encouragement to seek treatment should be
accompanied by a clear statement of the professional consequences if help is
not sought. Helpful and appropriate sanctions will vary with the individual, and the utmost sensitivity is required. Somehow this early intervention must connect with the life-sustaining side of the conflict present in the
suicidal patient. If this task can be accomplished, the chances of a successful
outcome increase.

The next step includes seeing a psychiatrist. As with any suicidal
patient, the diagnosis and the individual's personal resources will deter-

mine the management. Special considerations occur in the treatment setting because of the patient's professional status. Opinion varies in the literature about how much recognition should be given to the fact that the patient is a colleague. Sargent et al.[30] suggest that special treatment is necessary. They advocate "an attitude of collegial regard, which permits the doctor to sustain an already fragile self respect. The doctor's cooperation, which may depend on this attitude, is vital, because out-patient treatment may be the only kind the doctor will accept."

There is naturally a premium on techniques that build a strong therapeutic alliance. Such a bond can be instrumental in convincing the doctor not to practice or to enter a hospital as the situation warrants. Countertransference issues can be prominent when treatment involves a colleague; similarities in the patient's background and professional work can make over-identification a therapeutic hazard. Role expectations of doctor and patient must be clear but always supportive to the patient's impoverished self-esteem. Further, the treating psychiatrist should make no assumptions about the patient's knowledge about the illness, the therapeutic process, or psychopharmacological agents.

DEALING WITH THE IMPACT OF A SUICIDE

At times, despite recognition and treatment of the suicidal doctor, a fatality occurs. The following vignette provides an example of this unfortunate outcome:

> Trainees and staff in a psychiatric training program are shocked to hear that a resident, known to be having emotional difficulties and in treatment with an esteemed psychiatrist, has shot herself while parked in the therapist's driveway. Despite the doctor's impairment being both recognized and treated, the outcome was tragic.

A psychiatrist's committing suicide is deeply unsettling. The event is a grim reminder of the recent statistics that suggest a higher risk for members of that specialty. The suicide especially upsets those who fantasize that psychiatrists, by reason of their training, are better equipped to deal with emotional distress. Along with their sense of loss, colleagues may feel particular frustration that they were unable to assist one of their own, suffering from a condition about which they are the acknowledged experts.

Never easy, the task of informing patients of the physician's death is probably most difficult when the doctor is a psychiatrist. Several papers have recently dealt with the issues,[31-34] but are too varied to offer sensible generalizations about management. Opinions differ as to whether the therapist chosen to help the patient deal with the loss should be a friend of the dead psychiatrist or a less involved practitioner. Most writers agree that intervention should be early to help patients deal with the loss and reestablish a therapeutic relationship.

In addition to the fact that the doctor in the last vignette was a psychiatrist, that clinical example presents another disturbing piece of information: a physician's suicide can occur even when that person is in treatment. Those inevitable suicides that happen while the patient is in treatment leave the medical community reeling. It is sobering to realize that suicide cannot always be prevented, even when the patient is a doctor receiving proper treatment.

Whether the physician's suicide has occurred during treatment or suddenly without warning, the family, colleagues, and patients must contend with powerful emotions: sadness, guilt, anger, and perhaps shame. To assist the survivors, Shneidman[27] stresses the need for "postvention," a process in which they are encouraged to deal with their feelings about the loss. Specifically he defines it as activities that reduce the aftereffects of that "traumatic event in the lives of the survivors."

The responsibility for initiating such a therapeutic intervention naturally falls to a mental health professional, often a psychiatrist. Each case will require special consideration to determine the most appropriate mechanism by which to offer the "postvention." While the need will be greatest for the surviving family, colleagues who worked closely with the patient should have the chance to share their feelings as well. Experiences indicate that family members in particular find the postvention cathartic.

Cranshaw et al. recently underlined the severity of the impact on the family of physician suicides.[35] They convened a team to perform psychological autopsies on eight suicides which occurred in 1977 from a group of 40 Oregon physicians on probation. The team's recommendations included intervention as early as possible, strong but time-limited corrective action, and comprehensive mental health services for the survivors. They emphasized the need for help for the families of these troubled physicians. They urged the development of support groups as well as individual contact to help the families deal with their loss and sense of isolation. A strong plea was made for expanded research on the topic. They suggested that a national clearinghouse be developed under the auspices of the American Medical Association to facilitate the collection of reliable data on physician suicide.

In the past year, in fact, the AMA has set up a Physician's Mortality Study in conjunction with the American Psychiatric Association.[15] Currently a pilot project in five states, the group will perform psychological autopsies on physician suicides and a selection of suspicious deaths. The investigation will follow a carefully designed protocol that includes interviews with family as well as colleagues.

SUMMARY

The recent studies of physician suicide which suggest that the problem may be less dramatic statistically do not lessen the emotional trauma that all experience when their lives are touched by the grim event. While much remains to be learned about suicide in general, and physician suicide in particular, some specific suggestions are possible. The curriculum in medical schools should include programs that promote more self-awareness in future doctors of their emotional needs. If physicians cannot heal themselves, perhaps they can learn to recognize the need for assistance. Intervention (secondary prevention) requires that doctors must be able to believe that anyone can be suicidal, regardless of status. Professional roles should not prevent colleagues and friends from identifying prodromal clues. Finally, "postvention" (tertiary prevention) offers the survivors, be they family, colleagues, or patients, the opportunity to deal with the searing loss in a therapeutic way. The recently convened Physician's Mortality Study may provide insight and new approaches for dealing with this tragic consequence of physician impairment.

REFERENCES

1. Suicide among doctors, editorial: *Br Med J* 1:789–790, 1964.
2. Pasnau RO, Russell AT: Psychiatric resident suicide: An analysis of five cases. *Am J Psychiat* 132:402–406, 1975.
3. Rosen DH: Suicide rates among psychiatrists. *JAMA* 224:246–247, 1973.
4. Blachly PH, Osterud HT, Josslin R: Suicide in professional groups. *N Engl J Med* 268:1278–1282, 1963.
5. Craig AG, Pitts FN: Suicide by physicians. *Dis Nerv System* 29:763–772, 1968.
6. De Sole DE, Singer P, Aronson S: Suicide and role strain among physicians. *Am J Psychiat* 15:294, 1969.
7. Freeman W: Psychiatrists who kill themselves: A study of suicide. *Am J Psychiat* 124:846, 1967.
8. Suicides of physicians and the reasons, editorial: *JAMA* 41:263–264, 1903.
9. Knopf SA: Suicide among American physicians. *N Y State Med J* 117:84–87, 1923.
10. Dickinson FB, Martin LW: Physician mortality, 1949–1951. *JAMA* 162:1462, 1956.
11. Dublin LI, Spiegelman M: the longevity and mortality of American physicians. *JAMA* 134:1211, 1947.

12. Emerson H, Hughes HE: Death rates of male white physicians in the U.S. by age and cause. *Am J Public Health* 16:1088, 1926.
13. Von Brauchitsch H: The physician's suicide revisited. *J Nerv Ment Disorder* 162:40–45, 1976.
14. Bergman J: The suicide rate among psychiatrists revisited. *J Suicide Life Threat Behav* 9:219–226, 1979.
15. Steindler EM: Suicide in the Medical Profession: What the Research Does and Doesn't Show. Paper presented at the Mini-Conference on Physician Impairment, AMA Student Assoc. Annual Meeting, Houston, March 1981.
16. Rich CL, Pitts FN: Suicide by male physicians during a five-year period. *Am J Psychiat* 136:1089–1090, 1979.
17. Rose DH, Rosow I: Physicians who kill themselves. *Arch Gen Psychiat* 29:800–805, 1973.
18. Craig AG, Pitts FN: Suicide by physicians. *Dis Nerv System* 29:763–772, 1968.
19. Steppacher R, Mausner JS: Suicide in male and female physicians. *JAMA* 228:323–328, 1974.
20. Pitts FN, Schuller AB, Rich CL, et al: Suicide among U.S. women physicians. *Am J Psychiat* 136:694–696, 1979.
21. Robins E, Murphy GE, Wilkinson RH, et al: Some clinical considerations in the prevention of suicide based on a study of 134 successful suicides. *Am J Public Health* 49:888–899, 1959.
22. Pitts FN, Winokur G: Affective disorder: VII. Alcoholism and affective disorder. *J Psychiat Res* 4:37–50, 1966.
23. Zuk GH, Miller JB, Champagne EM, et al: Affective disorders and suicide in women physicians: Other views. *Am J Psychiat* 136:1604–1608, 1979.
24. Mausner JS, Steppacher RC: Suicide in professionals: A study of male and female psychologists. *Am J Epidemiol* 98:436–445, 1973.
25. Craig AG, Pitts FN: Suicide by physicians. *Dis Nerv System* 29:763–772, 1968.
26. Rich CL, Pitts FN: Suicide by psychiatrists: A study of medical specialists among 18,730 consecutive physician deaths during a 5 year period (1967–1972). *J Clin Psychiat* 41:261–263, 1980.
27. Shneidman FS: Suicide, in Freedman AM, Kaplan HT, Sadock BJ, (eds): *Comprehensive Textbook of Psychiatry II*. Baltimore, Williams & Wilkins Publishers, 1975, pp 1774–1785.
28. Pepitone-Arreola-Rockwell F, Rockwell D, Core N, et al: Fifty-two medical student suicides. *Am J Psychiat* 138:198–201, 1981.
29. Rockwell DA: Suicide in physicians. *Western J Med* 122:419–420, 1975.
30. Sargent DH, Jensen VW, Petty TA et al: Preventing physician suicide: The role of family colleagues and organized medicine. *JAMA* 237:143–146, 1977.
31. Ables BS: The loss of a therapist through suicide. *J Am Acad Child Psychiat* 13:143–152, 1974.
32. Chiles JA: Patient reactions to the suicide of a therapist. *Am J Psychiat* 28:115–121, 1974.
33. Graves JS: Adolescents and their psychiatrist's suicide: A study of shared grief and mourning. *J Am Acad Child Psychiat* 17:521–532, 1978.
34. Ballinger JC: Patients' reactions to the suicide of their psychiatrist. *J Nerv Ment Disorder* 166:859–867, 1978.
35. Crawshaw R, Bruce JA, Eraker PL, et al: An epidemic of suicide among physicians on probation. *JAMA* 243:1915–1917, 1980.

II

Medical School and the Impaired
Physician

5

Approaches to Prevention in Medical Education

BRIAN B. DOYLE AND DAVID W. CLINE

In recent years there has been a rapid growth of interest in and knowledge about impaired physicians, and about the emotional, professional, and financial expenses they incur. Increasingly, as these costs have become dearer, attention has turned to preventive as well as to therapeutic programs. This chapter focuses on preventive measures used in educational settings, in medical schools and in a continuing medical education course.

Although often advocated, prevention is rarely implemented in general medicine or in psychiatry. A notable exception in public health is vaccination such as against smallpox, which is clearly effective. Preventive measures are particularly difficult to evaluate in mental health programs, where the variables involved are so complex. Independent of the difficulties, however, we must still conceptualize and implement measures to prevent future impairment of physicians.

The theoretical framework for prevention in this chapter derives from the work of Caplan.[1] While there have been criticisms of his theoretical formulations, the framework provides a coherent way of thinking about the problems. According to Caplan, primary prevention involves lowering the rate of known cases of disorder in a population over a certain period by counteracting harmful circumstances before they have had a chance to produce other cases. Secondary prevention means shortening the duration of existing cases through early diagnosis and effective treatment. Tertiary prevention aims at reducing the community rate of defective functioning due to mental disorders. The princi-

BRIAN B. DOYLE • Department of Psychiatry and Behavioral Sciences, George Washington University School of Medicine and Health Sciences, Washington, D.C.   DAVID W. CLINE • Department of Psychiatry, University of Minnesota Medical School, and Coordinator of Medical Education, North Central Regional Medical Education Center, Minneapolis, Minnesota.

pal focus of tertiary preventive programs is to reduce the rate of residual disorders by restoring patients to their productive capacity. In this chapter each of these categories of prevention is discussed in theoretical terms and then compared with actual examples. Primary and early secondary prevention are emphasized since tertiary treatment networks have recently been surveyed by Fellows of the American Psychiatric Association.[2] While most of the examples are of primary and secondary prevention with medical students, one is included from a continuing medical education program for graduate physicians.

PRIMARY AND SECONDARY PREVENTION—MEDICAL SCHOOLS

The illustrative examples of primary and secondary prevention in the medical school setting are the products of telephone interviews by one of us (BBD) with key persons at 20 such institutions.[3] At each school contacted, a representative of the Department of Psychiatry was asked to identify the persons in the medical school most knowledgeable in this area. Up to three persons at a school were interviewed to fully investigate preventive activities. The interviews had three parts: an overview of the school, a structured set of questions about prevention, and a concluding discussion of themes and issues raised by the structured questions.

Primary Prevention

Primary prevention means lowering the incidence of disorders in a population. Effective primary prevention programs identify current harmful influences. They also locate environmental forces which support individual resistance and which enhance the population's resistance to further pathogenic experiences. Such programs require providing adequate physical, psychological, and sociocultural supplies to their populations. Primary prevention programs in a medical school setting require a locus for systematic planning for preventive mental health. Systematic planning includes research into environmental influences that operate for good and for ill, into assessment of student needs, and into methods of mobilizing resources. Effective primary prevention would require systematic attention to the psychological climate of the medical school in an official setting, such as an education evaluation committee or an office for student affairs. Primary prevention relies heavily on effective support networks, whether of faculty for students, of students for each other, or both.

In the schools included in this survey there was considerable skepticism about official systematic planning concerning student mental health needs. Of the 20 schools, 9 felt this did not take place; 5 schools did such work informally, and only 6 asserted that there was formal planning. Although there was general agreement about systematic planning, fiscal constraints and the press of other commitments kept it from being a high medical school priority.

Closely related to this research and planning function is assessment of student needs. It would be useful if at least one medical school committee officially included in its purview attention to quality-of-life issues for students. Most often this was not the case; of the 20 schools, 8 had committees with this function and 12 did not. At schools where committees did such work, it was part of a general school set towards students, such as the University of Minnesota, the University of Massachusetts, the University of California at Davis, Southern Illinois University, and Colorado. A promotions committee or its equivalent is the natural setting in which such issues surface. Typically, however, they do so in relation to individual student difficulties and there is little or no impact on the school's system as a whole.

The significant exception to this rule is the medical school at Stanford University. There the dean's office sponsored a committee on the Well-Being of the Medical Student and House Officer. The work of the committee culminated in a full report.[4]

A formal faculty advisor system is a familiar part of most medical schools, but one regarded with little enthusiasm. While only 4 schools had no such system, of the 16 schools with such a system only 5 rated it as working well. At the Medical School of the Uniformed Services, for example, each student has an advisor in his or her branch of service. Most schools regarded the system as highly variable, useful at best for specific career counseling, and having few preventive benefits.

Student-to-student advisory systems, while rarer, generate more enthusiasm where they do exist. As is characteristic of student-generated projects, their life is often relatively short; programs tend to be new. At the University of Massachusetts, for example, senior students for the first time in 1979 actively helped integrate freshmen into the school. At George Washington, there is a new peer-counseling system, with more advanced students providing advice, primarily about academic problems. At the University of Ohio (Toledo) there is also a peer-counseling system. In addition, senior students help younger ones choose clinical rotations and make career choices. Sophomores help orient freshmen. At the University of Cincinnati, a new peer-support system is run by sophomores for freshmen students.

Of the 20 schools surveyed, 10 formally sponsor support-oriented groups for students. At most of those, participation is voluntary. The University of Minnesota Medical School is unusual in requiring such an experience for all freshmen students (239 in toto). Groups of 10 freshmen meet for 2½–3 hours a week with a faculty advisor for their first academic quarter; the groups can elect to continue longer. Faculty and students at Minnesota feel that the groups are generally successful. Other schools have elective group experiences, some of which are led by members of the Department of Psychiatry, such as at Harvard, and some by members of the Department of Family Practice, such as at the University of New Mexico; in some, the leadership is from the dean's office and from varied departments, such as at George Washington School of Medicine. At the University of Ohio (Toledo), the transition from preclinical to clinical years is considered critical. That school formally sponsors small-group experiences for sophomores with role-playing and consultation by junior students, which continue until the students are established clinical clerks. There was a feeling, most strongly expressed by faculty at Harvard, that such groups have to be elective to be successful.

Representatives of 6 schools out of the 20 noted that small-group teaching in psychiatry and behavioral sciences has supportive functions. The respondents were ambivalent about this dual function, most considering the indirectly supportive group experience better than none. Courses about human development were convenient starting places for discussion of medical student life cycle issues in small group settings.

Some teachers were concerned that psychiatry small-group teaching can become almost exclusively process, with expression of student feelings at the expense of learning cognitive material. These teachers were wary of simply letting students ventilate. In their view, the small group becomes a lightning rod for dissatisfaction, with students displacing their anger and feelings about the medical school experience onto teachers and the subject matter of psychiatry. Other teachers felt that some expression of student feeling was inevitable. If handled properly, the discussion can be successfully incorporated in a larger exploration of the way psychiatrists operate, i.e., by acknowledging and expressing feeling while staying in professional role. In schools where there were no other settings available in which students could discuss their feelings, pressure could be considerable for small-group teaching in psychiatry to meet this need.

Factors involved in the outcome of faculty-run groups were complex. All who were interviewed agreed that success was markedly dependent on the personality of the group leaders. The capacity to lead well seemed highly individualistic and unrelated to medical specialty orientation. The interpersonal environment of the particular medical school was also important; faculty-led groups were most successful where students felt that teachers and administrators were interested in their well-being as well as in their academic progress. Where the faculty-led groups were successful, leaders and students became allies in the task of minimizing medical school stress and making it easier for students to learn and to grow. Successful group leaders found gratification from participating centrally in the human growth of future physicians. Through leading groups they provided students with experience and role models rather than with admonitions.

There was widespread dissatisfaction with traditional formal faculty–student advisory programs. Except in individual cases where the match was fortuitous, neither students nor faculty considered the results obtained worth the efforts expended. One school is considering abandoning its formal advisor system and instead deliberately matching individual or small-group needs as they arise with faculty with particular expertise or interest.

The issues are clearer about student-organized and student-run groups that have support functions. Medical school representatives were generally enthusiastic about such groups and tried to encourage them formally and informally. Fourteen of the schools surveyed had such groups. Several schools (i.e., Cincinnati, University of Massachusetts, Uniformed Services, Harvard, Marshall) noted the importance of women's student groups. A few schools (e.g., Uniformed Services, University of Texas at Houston, Cincinnati) emphasized the emergence of Christian student groups. Minority student groups, a natural focus of interest, varied widely in importance from school to school. They were essential at a school such as the University of Illinois, with a high percentage of minority students. At Yale, student support groups, labeled as such, have membership across the 4 years of medical school. Many student peer groups have support functions. These are explicit at some schools, such as in Yale's society for students interested in psychiatry, or in the group at the University of Massachusetts for students interested in family practice. A vigorous student council can itself be considered supportive. Student programs have taken different forms. At the University of Oregon, for example, students organized a humanistic medicine program in which group experiences are elective for a year or longer. Students at the University of Colorado systematically studied their clerkships and presented their findings to the medical school. After some resistance, changes recommended by the students were implemented.

Respondents by and large welcomed student groups wanting to

encourage student activities and responsibility. Experienced faculty and administrators were aware of the rising and ebbing of student interests. They emphasized riding with student enthusiasm, anticipating a cresting and slacking off of such activities.

There are other aspects of medical school life which apply to primary prevention, with orientation to medical school prominent among them. Among the approaches to orientation of the schools surveyed, the fullest was that at the Medical School of the Uniformed Services. Students enter basic training in their branch of service the summer before freshman year. The cohort in each class of each branch has been small. This results in natural group cohesion. The medical faculty organize the summer training so that the students develop an allegiance to the school as well as to their branch of the service. The result is a strong small-group bond which faculty find persists through the years at this new school.

At Marshall, in West Virginia, a new school with small class size, students spend orientation week in groups of four to six with individual faculty members. Much of the time is spent in touring, so that students get to know the service delivery catchment area. During this time the students begin to attach personally to faculty and to the school. Conceptually this can be viewed as a bonding experience, as a newborn optimally has with its parents.

Students at the University of Texas at Houston developed a week-end orientation program which was so successful that it is now being continued annually by the dean's office. Held away from the medical school site itself, it features small-group experiences and involves mingling more students and invited faculty with the newcomers.

Not all schools, however, have a glow of good feeling about orientation. At the University of New Mexico, for example, school representatives doubt that students hear messages about possible sources of difficulty and of potential help. Students are preoccupied with the excitement of starting medical school and enter with the familiar attitude that if anything is going to happen it will happen to someone else.

Caplan's[1] description of primary prevention includes providing adequate physical, psychological, and sociocultural supplies to a population. One example which neatly combines these occurs at Southern Illinois University School of Medicine, where there is an annual student loan fund evening. Only full-time faculty participate. Drinks and dinner precede an auction of goods donated by the faculty. The evening is a pleasant social occasion, and the money raised goes to a loan fund that provides for the kind of unforeseen emergencies that students inevitably encounter. The students get not only the money but tangible evidence of the faculty's capacity not just to care for them, but also to enjoy themselves. Contributions are, of course, tax deductible, so the only one who loses is Uncle Sam.

Secondary Prevention

Secondary prevention means reducing the disability rate due to a disorder by lowering its prevalence in the community. Early diagnosis and prompt treatment are essential. Diagnosis can be earlier if diagnostic tools are more effective, if one can alert potential patients and those in their social networks to earlier indications of disorder, and if one can motivate people to seek diagnostic investigations sooner. Facilities are necessary to investigate suspected cases promptly. Finally, treatment is more effective when diagnostic procedures lead rapidly to good therapeutic methods.

Making diagnostic tools more effective and available is a rational approach but one which is difficult to implement. In recent years legislation and a variety of other forces have prevented admission committees from inquiring about students with troubled past histories. Only 3 of the schools sampled actively inquired about these factors in the admissions process. At only 1 school of the 20, the University of Minnesota, was this inquiry rigorous. There, in addition to interviews by Admissions Committee members, all applicants take the Minnesota Multiphasic Personality Inventory (MMPI). If there is concern about the psychological stability of applicants, they are referred to a psychiatric consultant to the committee, whose recommendations markedly influence the decisions of the committee. With considerable experience in this role, the psychiatric consultant has been able to follow up on his early interventions and believes them to have been useful.

Minnesota is atypical. The more common attitude at most schools is that such investigation is flatly illegal. If anything, schools are being urged to make special provisions for students with a variety of handicaps.

At the other end of the spectrum is the medical school of the University of California at Davis. Administration and faculty there regard pre-admissions psychiatric screening as potentially harmful, since it could keep students who are potentially fine physicians out of medical school. We physicians need look no further than our own family and developmental histories to find support for the UC-Davis position!

Early-warning systems are imperative once the student is in medical school. At all schools surveyed, academic difficulty was an early warning which got prompt attention. Surprisingly few schools had formal study counseling programs which investigated the learning difficulties and proposed specific interventions for students. Many schools equated learning difficulties with emotional problems; all had systems designed to help academically failing students learn to cope.

How to detect or help the student who is doing adequately academically but not well otherwise is a thorny problem for most of the schools surveyed. Of the 20 schools surveyed, 13 had no system for finding or helping such students unless they identified themselves. Of the remaining 7, only 3 schools had systems which worked well: Emory, George Washington, and Minnesota were the exceptions. Officials at Minnesota credited a warm personal ambience with students as providing access. Built into the grading system in all courses in the clinical years at Emory is a component referred to as "suitability for medicine." This includes consideration of:

1. Concern for the welfare of patients
2. Concern for the rights of others
3. Responsibility to duty
4. Trustworthiness
5. Professional demeanor

The guidelines for each category are specific, as are the consequences of an unsatisfactory evaluation. Students are aware of the criteria and of the evaluation and appeal process.

George Washington Medical School's system for evaluation of nonacademic competence is complex, with careful consideration for the individual privacy of students. It requires a notification in writing to the associate dean for student affairs, which is kept confidential. The dean meets with the student whose nonacademic competence is in question and reviews the situation. That interview has several possible consequences. These include dropping the matter, recommending psychotherapy, or referring the student to a special sub-committee for further review. That sub-committee has numerous options, all of which are explicit and designed for the maximum protection of the student.

Another aid to early diagnosis is to provide the persons in the population with information about the early signs of problems. The rationale is that, given information about a disorder, persons will recognize it earlier in themselves and each other. This will lead to earlier referral and treatment. These assumptions, logical in themselves, are hard to test meaningfully in medical schools. The character of the interpersonal environment varies radically from school to school, from warmly supportive to isolated.

However, medical schools do transmit cognitive information well. As expected, the great majority of the schools sampled gave students facts about the subject areas related to impaired physicians: the stresses of professional life generally, typical medical personality patterns, mental illness and suicide, abuse of alcohol or other drugs, and marital and family problems. Table I summarizes the findings.

The curricular context for such information varies widely. Some schools give special lectures on the impaired or vulnerable physician while others have information relative to physicians emerge indirectly from courses on developmental issues or psychopathology. Yet another issue was the focus of such information; most respondents acknowledged that attention goes to the impaired or vulnerable physician, not the impaired or vulnerable medical student. If the focus is on the future physician rather than the student, then medical denial and avoidance is still served.

Medical educators know that simply to present cognitive material fails to guarantee that it is comprehended or used. Factual material about the impaired physician can be as abstract or as impersonal as the Krebs cycle, as readily memorized and easily forgotten. About a third of the schools sampled had found ways to present this material so that it would engage the students' emotions as well as their intellect. The medical schools at the University of Oregon and Southern Illinois University both use plays presented on slides, with a voice-over narrative. The plays illustrate the life of overworked and overstressed physicians. As such they supplement required reading and lecture material, powerfully stimulating discussion in small groups. At George Washington Medical School a panel of physicians and doctors' spouses discuss how their

Table I. Medical School Survey of Cognitive Information Concerning
Impaired Physicians

	Included in curriculum	
Subject area concerning physicians	Yes	No
General information about the stresses of a medical career	19	1
Abuse of alcohol or other drugs	18	2
Marital and family issues	16	4
Personality patterns of physicians	14	6
Suicide	14	6
Patterns of mental illness	12	8

experiences with problems such as alcoholism, overwork, and marital strain relate to their professional life. At Emory, four physicians with a history of substance-abuse problems make a presentation to the junior medical students. In Georgia, medical students participate electively in a sophisticated program for impaired physicians, learning especially about alcohol and other drug-abuse problems. Minnesota similarly has electives, popular with students, which allow them to work with physicians who have alcohol-related problems. Given the ubiquity of Alcoholics Anonymous and of physicians in AA groups, it is surprising that they generally interact so little with medical students. Comparatively speaking, alcoholic physicians are more organized and more available than doctors with other dysfunctions.

A good secondary prevention program will do more than dispense information about early warning signs of disorder. Another mainstay is to provide persons with whom troubled students can consult without labeling themselves as patients. Respondents at every school surveyed felt that such resources existed at their institutions. The helpers were numerous and varied, with individuals in the dean's office, the Department of Psychiatry, or other departments well known in their school for their availability and discretion. At schools such as UC-Davis, Minnesota, and George Washington there are elaborate measures to encourage students to seek help early, without negative sanctions. At all schools surveyed, respondents felt there were at least adequate provisions for early assistance.

Respondents at the large majority of schools sampled detailed explicit provisions for student confidentiality. At only one school was confidentiality not well defined or protected, and there it was a troublesome issue. At two other schools provisions about confidentiality were ambiguous, but the spokesmen asserted that operationally the system worked well. One of these schools was the Medical School of the Uniformed Services, where each student is considered to be on active military duty. Under these circumstances confidentiality is potentially a serious problem. To date the staff have successfully helped students get the help they need without adverse consequences. By and large the respondents felt that their institutions handle confidentiality well; it's just "not an issue," for example, at the University of North Dakota Medical School.

The final link in the chain of secondary prevention is prompt, effective treatment for diagnosed patients. Once again, representatives at all the schools surveyed felt that such was the case at their institution.

At virtually all the schools the finances for treatment costs were a problem, but there was a general conviction that students "somehow" get the treatment they need. Actual treatment systems vary widely and are the subject of an APA survey.[2]

Tertiary Prevention

Tertiary prevention is designed to reduce the rate of residual disorders by restoring patients to their productive capacity. This requires work both with affected persons and with the social systems they are to reenter, in this case medical students and medical schools. Although there was only general inquiry about this area the unanimous response of those questioned was that tertiary prevention goes well. Students generally have abundant personal resources, and medical schools generally are highly invested in returning dysfunctional trainees to full productive function. If anything, respondents at one or two schools were concerned that their institutions were too sympathetic to troubled students. According to the respondents in this sample, treatment and rehabilitation are far better handled than is prevention.

DISCUSSION

The rapid growth of interest in and study of the impaired physician are hopeful signs. From the information gathered, some recommendations emerge to maximize the value of medical student education to prevent the impairment of physicians.

The Uses of Orientation

Experiences at several medical schools surveyed (and others not included, such as at the University of Washington) confirm that orientation is potentially useful for prevention. During orientation a bond should develop between the school and the students, analogous to that between a newborn and its parents. At this time opportunities abound for positive informal interaction between students and faculty and administration, to foster an atmosphere of trust and cooperation. The examples cited in this chapter only represent what is being done and can be done.

Traditionally one thinks of "orientation" as being to the first year of medical school. The transition to the clinical years may well prove even more powerful in preventive terms. For many students medical school is a two-phase operation: the basic science years, which "you have to get through," and the clinical years, which are "the real stuff." An orientation to the clinical years, then, would reach students at their maximal affective engagement. One medical school (University of Ohio at Toledo) is exploring this transition in depth, seeking to maximize the students' growth at this time of emotional stress and intellectual overload.

The Uses of Support Groups

Again and again in respondents' replies hope was voiced for preventive benefits of small group experiences. Repetitively, psychiatric teachers alleged that such benefits occurred as a result of small-group teaching in their courses (allowing for the inevitable variability of group leaders). Although laudable, such indirect benefits are insufficient, and some medical schools successfully sponsor and run support-oriented groups.

Student-generated and run support groups are particularly powerful. Women's groups are increasingly numerous and important in medical schools. These can be expected to become even more significant as more women go into medicine.

There are beginning to be reports of the beneficial effects of support groups for house officers[5]; these clearly have enormous potential for medical students.

Foci for Preventive Intervention

There are now known areas of student difficulties where interventions are possible. It is surprising that so little happens, if the results of this survey are at all typical.

The first of these areas is difficulties in studying. Academic problems are sometimes simply academic problems. Good study counselors can investigate student learning difficulties, propose interventions, and follow up. The advantage of such a system is that students are not patients— they are students. If their grades improve their self-esteem rises, and the psychological benefits are great. If an academic problem is an emotional problem, that should become readily apparent in the process and a proper referral can be made. It is surprising that this relatively simple mechanism is so rare.

The other focus identified in this survey is more difficult to address. Workers at the University of California at Davis asserted that sexual problems are the major source of trouble for medical students, and that this is as true now as when it was first reported several years ago.[6] Sexual difficulties clearly can contribute to all of the ways in which physicians become impaired. Although many medical schools now have human sexuality programs, it is unclear how effectively these help students deal with their sexuality. If the UC-Davis experience is true of students at other schools, then there is an incentive to consider preventive interventions in this sensitive area. The subject deserves fuller exploration.

Uses of the Dean's Office

Effective medical school preventive programs are remarkably person-dependent. They generally rely heavily on a few key individuals in varied disciplines and in different departments. Increasingly they are in the dean's office. The responsibilties of a position such an an associate dean for student affairs are enlarging, if the schools surveyed are at all typical. Persons who have a special interest in preventive mental health are moving into such positions or are already in them, and that is another hopeful sign. The outstanding example in this survey is the Committee on the Well-being of Medical Students and House Officers, sponsored by the associate dean at Stanford.

Some assert that to incorporate preventive mental health measures formally in the dean's office is to undercut them, that there is a natural and inevitable gap between the students and the administration. According to this reasoning the stamp of official interest undercuts the best intentioned efforts.

In instances where the dean's office does not systematically address these issues, but only tolerates unofficial and individual efforts, then the institutional message is clear: these issues are not real or important, and they are not worth the investment of medical school resources. This parallels the attitude prevalent in organized medicine generally, at least until recently.

Beleaguered as they are with multiple demands in an era of dwindling resources, the deans understandably may be reluctant to invest in preventive mental health programs for students. Those who invest resources must do so against many other claims. Only when such programs become necessary for accreditation will medical schools systematically develop them. Prevention is a collective responsibility, and implementing this suggestion would lessen the burdens on those individuals who now shoulder a disproportionate amount of the preventive work.

Experience in large institutions teaches that formal policies and programs by themselves are insufficient. There will continue to be a need for the spontaneous and invaluable work of individuals and small groups among faculty, administration, and the students themselves.

PREVENTIVE INTERVENTIONS—CONTINUING MEDICAL EDUCATION

There has been little formal study of the possibilities of using Continuing Medical Education (CME) to prevent physicians from becoming impaired. The rapidly rising number of conferences devoted to the subject, however, reveals the growing interest. These are clearly based on the assumption that it will be helpful to provide physicians with cognitive knowledge and opportunities to exchange experiences.

One of the authors (DWC) conducted an experiment in prevention using a CME setting. He presented a 15-minute lecture describing physicians' problems with chemical dependency, especially alcohol. The lecture emphasized incidence, symptoms, confrontation techniques, treatment, and prognosis. It took place in a course about chronic obstructive lung disease and hypertension. Eighty-five physicians were in the audience. All men, they were from all specialties, from all over the United States, and ranged in age from 35 to 60. They held positions varying from heads of hospitals and medical societies to on-line practitioners.

There was an evaluation of the lecture's effectiveness at the end of the conference. Nine months later, a half-hour interview was structured to get data about the following topics: Did the subject remember the presentation? How did he feel about getting information he didn't bargain for? Had he changed his attitude toward chemical abuse? Had he changed his approach to patients, family friends, and employees? Had he changed his own drinking patterns? Ten control subjects who had not heard the 15-minute presentation were interviewed at follow up. The subjects were matched with the experimental subjects for age, position, and specialty. While the controls had not heard the lecture, they had had the same exposures to the news media, medical journals, and other casual educational interventions regarding chemical abuse that are available in the society at large.

Results

All the subjects filled out a questionnaire regarding the material of the conference at its close. Rating educational value on a 5-point scale, with 1 as excellent and 5 as poor, the general conference average was 1.8. Each lecture presentation was also evaluated; the 1.79 rating for the presentation on the problems of chemical abuse in the physician was about equal to other presentations. There were no critical comments about this unsolicited educational production.

Controls

The control subjects reported that they had made minor changes in their attitudes and clinical responses toward the chemically dependent person over the past 9 months. They reported that they were somewhat more aware of the problem of alcoholism and drug abuse. They were somewhat more optimistic about treatment but had not appreciably changed their approach to employees and family members. None of them said he changed his drinking pattern. A small but significant minority of the control group said that they had become more confrontive with their patients, their family members, and their employees on problems of alcoholism because of heightened awareness of it. However, they continued to see alcoholism as a moral weakness and admonished their affected affiliates as "helpless, spineless, and gutless." These physicians also watched their own drinking patterns. "If I think I am getting too dependent on my evening martinis, I stop drinking for two or three weeks to show that I can control it."

Experimental Group

All but 10% of the population interviewed remembered the lecture and its content 9 months later. None of these participants was offended by the presentation; all felt it was helpful in changing their attitudes and clinical practices regarding alcoholism. No experimental subject interviewed reported that his life had been radically changed as a result of a 15-minute educational intervention. However, most reported that this intervention was one in a series that highlighted the problems of alcoholism and drug abuse. It helped them further clarify their thinking and attitudes on this subject. The experimental subjects reported that they regarded alcoholism as a disease; through this and other educational experiences on chemical abuse they had become more sympathetic and understanding. The experimental subjects stated that they confronted patients in whom they suspected alcoholism more frequently than before the intervention. These physicians also felt a greater obligation to confront their friends, but none of them had done so directly. They did make indirect efforts, e.g., by talking with a spouse, or by sending an article on the complications of alcoholism to a friend in hopes that he "would get the message." The experimental subjects all reported an increase in confrontations with employees they felt had alcohol problems. Finally, the experimental group reported no significant change in their drinking patterns. However, they reported that they were more vigilant and thoughtful about their alcoholic intake patterns. These physicians were aware that they could become addicted to alcohol; they were also aware of their addiction to other substances such as coffee, cigarettes, and in some cases, to work and food. They reported that the educational intervention sensitized them to the possibility of other serious addictions.

CONCLUSIONS

This simple educational intervention, unsolicited by physicians participating in a continuing medical education course unrelated to alcoholism, had minor impact in changing patterns. However, it did tend to make an impact as part of a whole educational program about substance abuse. With other educational interventions on this subject, it reinforced ideas heard previously and brought to awareness concepts that were critical in assisting attitude change and building a knowledge base which may ultimately change personal behavior. Although statistical analysis of responses would not help, the trend is a positive one, and such educational efforts are to be encouraged, even if unsolicited by physician participants. Effort must be made to present the material by an authoritative presenter who introduces the subject with proper respect and regard for the audience. Finally, the relationship of this educational effort to the prevention of alcoholism is nowhere near the proven effectiveness of the Salk vaccine in preventing polio. At best it is comparable to that preventive admonition about polio: "Don't go swimming in the public swimming pool during August." We have a long way to go.

REFERENCE NOTES

1. Caplan G: *Principles of Preventive Psychiatry.* New York, Basic Books, 1964.
2. Newton P, Floyd R, Valdes U, et al: American Psychiatric Association/National Institutes of Mental Health Study of Medical Students' Mental Health Services, 1979.
3. Schools and persons contacted include:
   (1) University of Arizona School of Medicine; Stephen Scheiber, M.D.
   (2) University of Cincinnati School of Medicine; Jerald Kay, M.D., Director, Medical Student Education in Psychiatry
   (3) University of Southern California School of Medicine; Sherwyn Woods, M.D., Director of Psychiatric Residency and of psychotherapy program for medical students
   (4) University of Colorado School of Medicine; Steven P. Dubovsky, M.D., Director of Medical Student Education in Psychiatry
   (5) Emory University School of Medicine; John Griffin, M.D., Director, Medical Student Education in Psychiatry

(6) George Washington University School of Medicine; Robert Keimowitz, M.D., Associate Dean for Student Affairs, and Winfield Scott, Ph.D., Associate Dean for Education

(7) Harvard University School of Medicine; Carol Nadelson, M.D., Coordinator of Medical Student Teaching, Beth Israel Hospital

(8) University of Illinois School of Medicine; Sara Charles, M.D., Associate Director, Medical Student Education

(9) Marshall University School of Medicine; Mildred Mitchell-Bateman, M.D., Chairman, Department of Psychiatry

(10) University of Massachusetts (Worcester) School of Medicine; Alan J. Barnes, M.D., Coordinator, Medical Student Education in Psychiatry

(11) University of Minnesota School of Medicine; George Williams, M.D., Associate Dean for Student Affairs, and Pearl Rosenberg, Ph.D., Office for Student Affairs

(12) University of New Mexico School of Medicine; Scott Obenshain, M.D., Assistant Dean for Undergraduate Education, and Donald West, M.D., Director of Undergraduate Education in Psychiatry

(13) University of North Dakota School of Medicine; Russell M. Gardner, M.D., Chairman, Division of Psychiatry

(14) Ohio (Toledo) School of Medicine; Lane Gerber, Ph.D., Associate Dean for Student Affairs

(15) University of Oregon School of Medicine; Richard Angell, M.D., Director, Student Mental Health Service

(16) University of Southern Illinois School of Medicine; Terry Travis, M.D., Acting Chairman, Department of Psychiatry

(17) Stanford University School of Medicine; John Steward, M.D., Associate Dean for Student Affairs, and Harvey Weinstein, M.D., Psychiatrist, Student Health Service

(18) University of Texas (Houston) School of Medicine; Richard du Vaul, M.D., Associate Dean for Student Affairs, and Sidney Zisook, M.D., head of Medical Student Education in Psychiatry

(19) Medical School of the Uniformed Services; John Duffy, M.D., head of Medical Student Education in Psychiatry

(20) Yale University School of Medicine; Marshall Edelson, M.D., Director, Medical Student Education in Psychiatry; John Docherty, M.D., and James Charney, M.D., Department of Psychiatry.

4. Report of the Dean's Committee on the Well-Being of the Medical Student and House Officer, Stanford University School of Medicine, 1980.
5. Siegel B, Donnelly JC; Enriching personal and professional development: The experience of a support group for interns. *J Med Educ* 53:908–914, 1978.
6. Wood SB: Sexual problems of medical students. *Med Aspects Hum Sexuality,* 6:66–85, 1972.

6

The Medical School Admissions Committee
A Preventive Psychiatry Challenge

STEPHEN C. SCHEIBER

Many medical students who sought psychiatric help had personality problems before entering medical school and the major cause of mal-adaptation was "the personality they brought with them," according to Hunter et al.[1] The study of psychiatric illness in medical students by Pitts et al. demonstrated a high correlation with family histories positive for psychiatric illness.[2] Modlin and Montes, in their study of physician addicts, and Vaillant et al., in their work on psychological vulnerabilities, point to early childhood factors that influence the need for psychiatric care.[3,4] Blachly et al. describe the physician at risk for suicide as "competitive, compulsive, individualistic, ambitious, a graduate of a high prestige school, one who had mood swings, had problems with drugs, or alcohol, a non-lethal annoying physical illness, and one who may feel a lack of restraint by society."[5] These risk factors are discussed in Chapter 1, Emotional Problems of Physicians: Nature and Extent of Problems.

Goodwin, in his studies on familial alcoholism,[6,7] determined that children of alcoholics are particularly vulnerable to alcoholism. "Sons of alcoholics were about four times more likely to become alcoholics than were sons of non-alcoholics. About 30% of daughters of alcoholics had been treated by age 32 for depression compared to about 5% of the control group. Familial alcoholism is characterized by (1) a family history of alcoholism; (2) early onset of alcoholism. The sons of alcoholics were alcoholics by their late 20's; (3) severe symptoms requiring treatment at an early age; and (4) absence of other conspicuous psychopathology.[7]

STEPHEN C. SCHEIBER • Department of Psychiatry, University of Arizona College of Medicine, Tucson, Arizona. Revised and reprinted with permission from the *Psychiatric Forum*, Spring 1976.

According to Pepitone-Arreola-Rockwell et al., female medical students are 3–4 times more at risk for suicide than their agemates in the general population.[8] Epstein et al. judge that physician suicide may be predicted based on the medical student's characteristics.[9] Paffenbarger et al. address the issue of chronic illness as a precursor of suicide.[10,11]

These studies point to the need for medical school admissions committees to review carefully high-risk candidates as well as those with gross deviations at the time candidates are being considered for admission. Talbott and Michels advise that one of the roles of a psychiatrist on an admissions committee is to use his expert knowledge as a consultant to "assess whether an applicant with an illness or disability will be able to handle the stress of medical school and the medical profession."[12] Fifty percent of medical school admissions committees requested psychiatric consultation when a candidate had a history of mental illness, according to Silver et al.[13] The review of high-risk candidates is important in spite of the caution by Shapiro et al., "it is not yet practical to talk of fool-proof screening of medical school candidates, as only the grossest kinds of disorders can be detected."[14]

Waring's careful review of psychiatric illnesses in physicians mentions the difficulties with screening the population at risk and identifies the responsibility of selection committees.[15]

Garfinkel and Waring, in discussing emotional problems in psychiatric residents, also conclude that the "major factor in pychiatric disturbance is the personality of the individual." They caution that psychometric screening tests may be unreliable in individual cases. Emotionally disturbed residents in their studies scored higher on the neurotic scale of the Eysenck Personality Inventory and on the scales for measuring depression, isolation, and confusion of the MMPI compared to their colleagues. "Their interests more closely resembled bankers than other psychiatrists or physicians."[16]

THE CURRENT STATE OF THE ART

Currently admission committees rely on grade-point scores in colleges and universities, medical aptitude tests, letters of recommendation from undergraduate faculties, personal interviews of candidates, application data, and health questionnaires to assess candidates for medical schools. The emphasis placed on each data source will vary among schools. The first four items are usually given the most weight, in varying proportions, compared to the latter two.

Although health questionnaires of candidates could serve as useful sources of data, this author's experience on an admissions committee has been that they are often filled out by busy family physicians who, if they do more than the perfunctory, use this vehicle as much, if not more, as a reference letter in support of the candidate than as a comprehensive health document. Similarly, the reports of untrained, voluntary interviewers in the admissions process leads to nondiscriminatory, uninformative, and psychologically naïve data that rarely include any high-risk information, and sometimes miss gross deviation. Such interview reports add little to the consideration of psychological vulnerabilities in assessing individual candidates. Letters of recommendation from undergraduate college faculties seldom include anything but laudatory comments, frequently supporting the high academic achievements that already can be deduced from viewing the candidate's grades. Thus admissions committees can easily be lulled into dealing principally with such "hard data" as medical college aptitude tests and grade-point averages which give comfort to those faculty members who give special credence to these numbers as evidence of the student's ability to pass their courses.

RECOMMENDATIONS

In spite of the cautionary remarks that only the grossest deviation can be detected at the time of the medical school admission interviews, and given the limitations of generalizing from small skewed samples of deviant populations, it appears that admissions committees can pay more attention to studying high-risk psychiatric populations in considering applicants to medical schools.

The following data should be gathered on all medical student applicants:

1. A comprehensive three-generation history of drug taking, alcoholism, and emotional and mental illnesses (with a separate statement on mood swings, depression, and suicide for purposes of emphasis). This should include parents, grandparents, their siblings, and the candidate and his siblings.[2,6,17]
2. A childhood history of early disturbances such as colic and enuresis, and chronic childhood illnesses.[3]
3. A description of mother–child relationships from infancy to present.[4]

4. A statement of father–child relationships from infancy to present.[4]
5. A description of the home atmosphere in growing up.[4]
6. Recreational, avocational, peer group interests and activities.[4]
7. Relationships with significant others.[4]
8. Marital histories and description of relationships.[4]
9. Description of relationships with candidate's children.[4]
10. If unmarried, discussion of future marital plans.[18]

These data ideally should be obtained from four different sources. First, the applicant should be asked to supply the data as part of his application. Second, the family doctor, who may indeed know a three-generation medical history, should fill out a comprehensive family history form. Third, the undergraduate school should be asked to supply data regarding family, social, and psychological health of the candidate's college years.

Most important, the medical school interviewers should have available to them any data suggesting the presence or absence of psychological vulnerabilities from the other three sources. Even in the absence of data from the other three sources, at least one-third of the interview should be devoted to exploring this area. In order for this to de done within the time constraints of interviewing, gifted, experienced interviewers must be used.

The last requisite may present the greatest limitation in the entire process. Admission interviewing often is one of the many competing voluntary functions of a busy faculty, and has few rewards other than personal, altruistic ones. Rarely is any recognition given to this important and, in rare cases, potentially lifesaving function, other than a perfunctory letter of recognition from the dean's office. If no other rewards are possible within a medical school, then deans may be advised to hire and pay skilled interviewers.

Upon reviewing the health data, admissions committees should have guidelines to suggest which are the vulnerable candidates. When there is doubt about an individual, then an interview by a psychiatrist should be obtained and risk factors further evaluated. High-risk candidates should be identified and the nature of the risk shared with the admissions committee. As Talbott and Michels point out, such information tends to work in favor of the candidate rather than against him. The psychiatrist should be asked for an opinion regarding prognosis for the candidate.[12]

DISCUSSION

It is not sufficient simply to collect this data. Admissions committees should have the benefit of a psychiatrist to interpret psychological and/or high-risk data so that intelligent use of this information can be incorporated into the decision-making process. In spite of the caution that good doctors can come from troubled families, they are nevertheless in a higher risk category. Likewise, a candidate who grows up in a sea of psychosis, drug taking, alcoholism, depression, suicide, and/or other psychopathologies is more vulnerable to mental illness than his counterpart with similar medical college aptitude test scores and grade-point average who grew up in a psychologically healthy environment.

Also, since trouble with drugs, psychiatric hospitalizations, and suicides most frequently comes to attention when the physician is in his 40's, admissions committees might decide that it is too early to determine future behaviors. In an absolute sense they would be correct. However, psychiatry has demonstrated that behavior patterns can be studied. Even knowledge that one suicide attempt does not confer immunity against future attempts, but enhances risk, may alert committee members to evaluate suicide data along with aptitude test scores and grade-point averages. This is only one illustration of how such data may be useful.

Psychological vulnerability histories and psychological assessments of individual candidates give important data for medical school admissions committees to consider. Appraisal of the data in the admissions process is not meant to replace secondary prevention methods through education of physician students as to the high risk of the profession he is entering nor to discourage psychotherapy for physician students and/or graduate doctors.

Indeed, Talbott and Michels point out that high-risk candidates who are admitted may need support when special difficulties arise in medical school.[12] This would be consistent with the legislation protecting the rights of the handicapped.[19] The identification of high-risk physicians enlarges the responsibilities of hospital staffs, medical societies, or spouse clubs for providing legitimate, improved therapy and support or counsel to disturbed physicians. Knowledge of high-risk groups will not prevent future doctors from developing emotional disturbance. The data will be most useful if they are used in a longitudinal study of populations considered high risk, controlled with those considered as low risk for both populations accepted to medical school and those not. In 20–30 years admissions committee members can compare outcomes of those accepted to medical school with those not accepted, and it can then be determined whether a career in medicine contributed to psychiatric morbidity and mortality. Committees will know whether they helped to avert a suicide. Preservation of one life is worth the effort!

REFERENCES

1. Hunter RCA, Lorenz JG, Schwartzman AE: Nosophobia and hypochondriasis in medical students. *J Nerv Ment Disorder* 139:147–152, 1964.
2. Pitts FN Jr, Winokur G, Steward MA: Psychiatric syndromes, anxiety symptoms and response to stress in medical students. *Am J Psychiat* 118:333–340, 1961.
3. Modlin HC, Montes A: Narcotic addiction in physicians. *Am J Psychiat* 121:358–366, 1964.
4. Vaillant GE, Sobowale NC, McArthur C: Some psychological vulnerabilities of physicians. *N Engl J Med* 287:372–375, 1972.
5. Blachly PH, Disher W, Roduner G: Suicide by physicians. *Bull Suicidology,* NIMH, Dec: 1–18, 1968.
6. Goodwin DW: Familial alcoholism. Paper presented to APA, New Orleans, May, 1981.
7. Goodwin DW: Alcoholism and heredity: A review and hypothesis. *Arch Gen Psychiat* 36:57–61, 1979.
8. Pepitone-Arreola-Rockwell F, Rockwell D, Core N, et al: Fifty-two medical student suicides. *Am J Psychiat* 138:198–201, 1981.
9. Epstein L, Thomas CB, Shaffer J, et al: Clinical prediction of physician suicide based on medical student data. *J Nerv Ment Disorder* 156:19–29, 1973.
10. Paffenbarger R, King S, Wing A: Chronic disease in former college students: LX. Characteristics in youth that predispose to suicide in later life. *Am J Public Health* 59:900–908, 1969.
11. Paffenbarger R, Asnes D: Chronic diseases in former college students: III. A precursor of suicide in early and middle life. *Am J Public Health* 56:1026–1036, 1966.
12. Talbott JA, Michels R: The role of psychiatrists in the medical school admissions process. *Am J Psychiat* 138:221–224, 1981.
13. Silver LB, Nadelson CC, Joseph EJ, et al: Mental health in medical student applicants: The role of the admissions committee. *J Med Educ* 54:534–538, 1979.
14. Shapiro ET, Pinsker H, Shale JH: The mentally ill physician as practitioner. *JAMA* 232:725–727, 1975.
15. Waring EM: Psychiatric illness in physicians: A review. *Compr Psychiat* 15:519–530, 1974.
16. Garfinkel PE, Waring EM: Personality, interests and emotional disturbances in psychiatric residents. *Am J Psychiat* 138:51–55, 1981.
17. Pescor MJ: Physician drug addicts. *Dis Nerv System* 3:2–3, 1942.
18. Steppacher R, Mausner J: Suicide in male and female physicians. *JAMA* 238:323–328, 1974.
19. Office of the Secretary, Department of Health, Education and Welfare: Rules and regulations on nondiscrimination on basis of handicap. *Federal Register,* March 4, 1977, pp 22676–22701.

7

Medical Student Stress, Adaptation, and Mental Health

CAROL C. NADELSON, MALKAH T. NOTMAN, AND
DAVID W. PREVEN

With the growth of interest in the problem of the impaired physician and concerns about the origins and possible preventive approaches, attention has been focused on the mental health of medical students, and more specifically on their psychological vulnerabilities. Medical training shares many characteristics with other graduate and professional programs. There are, however, some specific and unique features: the length, rigidity, and intensity of the training period from the beginning of medical school through residency is unequalled in other professional or graduate programs. Although other educational programs may span the same number of years, they do not involve the same total and inflexible commitment during those years.[1,2,3]

The competitiveness of the medical school atmosphere, as well as the academic pressures, are experienced as stressful by most students. Although on the whole these students adapt, many pay a high price.[4-10] For some, conflicts engendered in this process result in somatic or emotional symptoms including depression, anxiety, self-doubt, academic difficulties, or family problems.[6,7,11-21] Other students find that their preexisting problems worsen. Still others are confronted with crises in their families or difficulties in interpersonal relationships.

Medical school is also stressful because students often find themselves unable to maintain old relationships or make new ones. Time and energy are at a premium, and those outside of their immediate environ-

CAROL C. NADELSON • Department of Psychiatry, Tufts University School of Medicine, Boston, Massachusetts   MALKAH T. NOTMAN • Department of Psychiatry, Tufts University School of Medicine, Boston, Massachusetts   DAVID W. PREVEN • Department of Psychiatry, Albert Einstein College of Medicine of Yeshiva University, Bronx, New York.

ment may not understand the pressures they experience. Students find that their friends either leave them or are not sympathetic to their preoccupations. Their families are often distant or alienated. They even lose interest in people and activities that had been rewarding in the past. At times friends and relatives make new demands that the students provide information and act "like a doctor," a shift for which the student is unprepared.

The medical student must also acquire and integrate a large body of medical information and develop the complex medical skills that transpose someone who feels inept into a physician. Simultaneously, the consolidation of personal identity and further separation from family also occur. Like others of their age, medical students continue to deal with these developmental issues, including the shift from a position of dependency on others, e.g., parents, to greater independence. They must also begin to assume major responsibilities for patients as well as for themselves and their families.[22] These factors, plus individual personality traits and capacities, are important in determining how students adapt and what difficulties they encounter.

What is known about the emotional health and adaptation of medical students? What psychological assessments of the 60,000 students currently enrolled in medical school have been made? How often do they seek psychiatric consultation and for what kinds of problems? How do requests for psychiatric help relate to the actual stress experienced? How do medical students compare with other students with regard to psychiatric problems?

One way to answer these questions is to examine some crude measures of psychopathology, e.g., rates of suicide, psychiatric hospitalization, and drug and alcohol abuse. Another approach is to attend to more complex manifestations of stress, such as attrition rate or academic performance. Finally, we can look at the perceptions that medical students have of their experiences and the kinds of resources they seek. These perceptions change throughout the 4 years of school as developmental tasks are or are not met successfully.

While a strict view of the prevalence of particular mental illnesses can facilitate planning for necessary resources, it can also be used to avoid the complex and multi-faceted problems brought by students, which cause them distress and may or may not diminish their observed functioning.

Students reach out for help in a variety of ways. This occurs not necessarily because they are ill, but because they are stressed. The solutions they seek are related to the help available, as well as to their own personal styles and value systems. This chapter will review the limited data available on prevalence of psychopathology in selected samples of medical students' mental health resources, using illustrative clinical material.

MEASURES OF PSYCHOPATHOLOGY

Suicide

The occurrence of this event in young, highly selected trainees is tragic. Controversy about it in the literature followed Simon's 1968 report[9] of a 20-year follow-up of medical student deaths; he asserted that between 1947 and 1967 suicide was the second most common cause of death among medical students. This occurred at a time when there was a 24% increase in the same age group in the general population. A recent study by Everson and Fraumeni,[23] however, indicates that the incidence is in fact *less* than that for the same age group in the general population.

In 1973 Epstein reported on longitudinal data collected on graduates of Johns Hopkins Medical School from 1948 through 1964.[24] She was able to predict later suicide on the basis of personality data from tests given during medical school. She found that those who committed suicide had poor self-images, low self-esteem, depression, anger, and fear. Although the number was small, thus making interpretation difficult, the data certainly suggest that it is possible to identify those who are more likely to suffer emotional problems. This concurs with Simon, who points out that those students who committed suicide had a history of irregular progress through medical school.

Psychiatric Hospitalization

There are currently no specific studies on the incidence of psychiatric hospitalization among medical students. While criteria for hospitalization are variable, Thomas's research provides some useful information on incidence.[10] Of the 1337 students her group studied, 11 students required psychiatric hospitalization. Over the 16 years of the study this would result in an approximate rate of hospitalization of one student each 18 months. While this rate corresponds to the experience at other institutions, more systematic and current data are needed describing the rate and criteria for student psychiatric hospitalization.

Drug and Alcohol Abuse

The literature in this area also does not provide conclusive data. One self-report survey of 172 students at a midwestern school, using criteria such as drinking while studying, "passing out after drinking," using alcohol therapeutically, and receiving treatment for drinking, reported that 10% could be identified as problem drinkers.[25] Clearly this survey also needs to be replicated at other institutions. Designing a more representative sampling system and defining clearer criteria for alcohol abuse are necessary future tasks.

There has been attention also to nonmedical use of drugs among medical students. The use of marijuana, especially in the early 1970s, seemed to parallel its use generally among young adults. Mechanick et al. reported that from 1970 to 1972, although there was an increase in the number of students using cannabis, there was a marked decline in the frequency of use among those studied.[26] Lipp et al. found that the use of marijuana was strongly influenced by geographical region, varying from 17% at one school to 70% at another.[27] In one of the few studies comparing medical students with law students at the same university, Slaby et al. found no difference in marijuana use.[28] They also noted that approximately 7% of both law and medical students reported using amphetamines at least once.

These studies all attempt to assess the prevalence of drug or alcohol use in a sample of the student population. Another approach would be to identify the extent of drug or alcohol problems in students seeking psychiatric treatment. In those reports that list such diagnoses, substance abuse was one of the least often mentioned.[8,29] Of course, students may be hesitant to seek treatment for a problem that, if discovered, would be detrimental to their career. Confidentiality is clearly an important consideration in a student's decision to request help.

Attrition Rates

If the objective of admission committees is to choose students who will complete the training program, they are currently achieving that goal with remarkable success. The present highly competitive selection process succeeds in eliminating those who cannot survive the training ordeal. Overall attrition rates for the years 1975–1978 have been remarkably low, less than 2% (excluding those who transfer or withdraw for advanced study).[30] Even if one agrees that emotional stress is a reason for dropping out, it would be erroneous to conclude that completion of the training indicates absence of emotional turmoil. There have been several reports indicating that in both college and medical school academic success can occur despite significant psychopathology.[5,31] The success of the process of selecting individuals with the intellectual and psychological resources to complete their studies is noteworthy, since admissions committees know relatively little about a prospective student's mental health. A recent survey, which reported data from 63% of the nation's medical schools, indicated that only one-third of the schools asked about previous or current psychiatric illness or treatment at a time when there were no real constraints against doing this.[32] With current legislation preventing discrimination against otherwise qualified applicants because of physical or emotional handicaps, it is less likely that information about prior difficulties will be available. As a result there are likely to be more medical students entering schools with a prior history of emotional problems. This is especially important in view of the data suggesting that previous life history is an important factor in the subsequent development of emotional problems, alcoholism, and addictions in physicians.[33-35] Furthermore, Hunter et al. reported that students whose emotional problems antedated medical school required more hours of treatment and had less satisfactory results.[36] This finding must receive attention in future planning. One must also remember that prior psychotherapy alone does not necessarily tell much about emotional problems, since therapy may be more available and less stigmatizing in some geographic areas or schools than in others.

INCIDENCE OF PSYCHOPATHOLOGY

There have been some attempts at systematic research on the incidence of psychopathology in medical students. A recent preliminary survey indicated that about 20% of the 53 responding schools had some kind of personality assessment after admission.[29] Only one school had a routine, but voluntary, psychiatric interview after admission.

In the early 1960s Pitts et al. interviewed a random sample of a medical sophomore class and reported that 6 out of 40 were "psychiatrically ill."[37] (Three students were diagnosed as having bipolar affective illness, one as having an anxiety neurosis, one as chronically alcoholic, and one psychiatrically ill but undiagnosed.) He also noted that anxiety symptoms did not increase appreciably in the "psychiatrically ill" during exam periods. Furthermore, those with such illnesses also reported a higher incidence of psychiatric disorder in family members.

Golden et al. compared 50 medical students with 50 students selected for their "normal" Minnesota Multiphasic Personality Inventories (MMPI).[38] Using the MMPI scores as criteria, 25 of the medical students and only 3 of the "normals" were considered to have significant psychopathology. Half of those medical students (13 of 25) were diagnosed as having characterological problems.

Additional reports deal more with psychological and personality traits than with psychopathology. Schlageter and Rosenthal[39] and Keniston[40] have commented on the frequently observed medical student personality characteristics of repression, isolation, and high need for achievement and productivity. In a comprehensive review of the medical student's psychosocial attributes, McGuire concluded that the students were able to deal realistically with an environment that is "demanding and threatening"; the major source of threat is uncertainty of success in a profession in which so much has been invested.[6] Especially in the preclinical phase, the "war with faculty" over what should be learned emerged as a major stress.

The impact of a particular stress, of course, depends on the resources and interests of the student. In one study, Schwartz et al. compared a group of students who said that they would choose a career in the humanities if they had not chosen medicine ("artistic-literary") with those who would choose science ("physician-surgeon").[41] They measured disillusion with the choice of medicine in the fourth year. As might be anticipated, 29% of the "artistic-literary" group but only 14% of the "physician-surgeon" group expressed regrets about choice of career and the medical school experience. This is, of course, at the point where students have not yet had the opportunity to shape their own careers and when they are experiencing maximal demands of their clinical rotations. Schwartz and colleagues also noted a tendency for more "artistic-literary" students than "physician-surgeon" students to enter psychotherapy.

Edwards and Zimet reported that students with the greatest personality resources showed the least amount of stress-related anxiety.[13] They listed the problems of medical students as separation anxiety, homosexual anxiety, depression, depersonalization, and fear of failure. Coburn and Jovacas also emphasized the stressful nature of the academic pressures, especially for students who were not part of the mainstream of medical students, including those from the lower social class, unfamiliar with the city, female, or minority students.[42]

USE OF MENTAL HEALTH RESOURCES

While visits to student health facilities are often used as an index of need, Reifler and Babineau emphasized that this is a poor measure of incidence of illness because of the large number of factors which determine utilization.[43] These include availability, accessibility, and acceptability of treatment. In addition, the visibility and reputations of therapists and their departments are important.[44] Prompt response to the student's request for evaluation and a staff that is viewed as warm, competent, and informed about medical student life promote a good reputation.

The visibility of the clinic staff as faculty members is also important.[44] The opportunity to observe the psychiatrist as a knowledgeable and sensitive clinician will often encourage a student in need to seek consultation. Factors which apear to increase utilization of services are probably related more to attitudes and understanding than to illness. Sex, religion, class, geography, and age, as well as available supports, are also important determinants. More likely to seek help are women, Jews, and nonreligious students, students from professional and managerial families, students from urban environments, younger students, and those without organizations and supports more than students who are socially active.[45]

In a survey of medical student mental health services more than 90% of respondents provided some form of mental health care.[29] The use of services by 10%–25% of the student enrollment is comparable to that in other graduate schools. In a 1-year survey, 20% of students from the Harvard Graduate School of Arts and Sciences and 10% of those from the Harvard Business School sought psychiatric consultation.[46,47]

A number of reports provide an overview of student mental health needs and services.[5,11,15,29,36,44,48] Although there are some exceptions, an overall average of 10%–25% of students seek psychiatric consultation or treatment. The actual figure is probably higher because many authors do not report on students seeing a private psychiatrist. The largest number appear to seek help during the first year. Thereafter there is variability from school to school. Self-referral is the most common method of obtaining treatment. There is controversy, however, about whether the self-referral reflects the student's own enlightened appreciation of what psychiatry can offer or, as some have suggested, simple "benign neglect" by the medical school faculty.[43]

There is also diversity of opinion over what role the medical school plays in precipitating the need for treatment. At McGill, Hunter reported that 40% (21 of 53) of the student patients had psychiatric problems prior to admission.[36] He discovered that another 26% entered treatment because of stresses secondary to medical school, and over a third (18 of 53) sought help for factors unrelated to academic work.

Adsett reported that 13% of the medical students at the University of Oklahoma received counseling for psychological problems each year, and that a higher percentage were seen for somatic complaints in which emotional conflicts were etiological to a significant degree.[11] He cited three basic problem areas. First was developmental issues related to the adjustments of late adolescence and early adulthood, including concerns about identity, conflicts around conformity versus rebellion, and reality versus idealism. The second problem area was the activation of long-standing, latent intrapsychic conflicts. These involved issues of dependency and separation, often manifested in concerns about financial dependence and in problems with authority figures. Sexual adequacy was also a frequent issue. The third major area was the response to the educational process and the school milieu.

The manifest symptoms Adsett found included anxiety, depression, hypochondriasis, and personality disorders (obsessive-compulsive, passive-aggressive, and schizoid). He found that both sociopathy and psychosis were uncommon. He also noted that psychological problems adversely affected academic performance.

There are, however, conflicting reports about the association of academic achievement and emotional symptoms. In one study, a comparison of admission grade-point average (GPA) and Medical College Admission Test (MCAT) scores failed to distinguish students who later performed poorly because of emotional problems.[36]

Lief et al. reported that students requesting psychiatric consultation came largely from the top and bottom third of the class.[5] Johnson and Hutchins,[16] on the other hand, found that twice as many students who were unsuccessful academically reported emotional difficulties than those who were successful, and Golden et al. noted poorer academic performance in students receiving psychiatric treatment.[38] They added that those students with extraordinarily high MCAT scores were able to compensate for their psychological difficulties, and thus were less likely to show poor performance. A fair conclusion about school performance and psychiatric treatment may be that poor academic work is often associated with emotional difficulty, but a good record does not guarantee emotional well-being.

BEYOND THE PSYCHIATRIC CLINIC: APPROACHES TO PREVENTION

For most students, the stresses experienced in the training program do not result in requests for psychiatric consultation.[13,42,49] In the preclinical phase, the realization that one can no longer master all the course material is often a profound blow to self-esteem. Students whose self-image relied totally on academic achievement are especially vulnerable to depression.[44,45] Successful adaptation in the first two years requires that the students modify previous highly perfectionistic standards of achievement. They must accept that they are now in a group of academic superstars. This must be accomplished in an environment in which faculty expectations are often unrealistic as well as vaguely defined. As Rosenberg states, "the violence done to the self-image of the medical student is the most serious consequence of his educational program."[50]

For many students, the stresses experienced during the clinical phase are less disabling. While long hours, work with critically ill patients, and gradual acceptance of responsibility for patient care all produce stress, they are demands that most students anticipated. The most commonly mentioned stress during the early clinical years involves interactions with attendings, initial attempts at case presentations, the questioning process on rounds, and unsatisfactory working relationships with house officers.[51]

For most students, stress can be handled with problem-oriented, time-limited interventions. Reports in the literature suggest that a variety of therapeutic techniques have been successful. These include support groups,[52] peer-counseling programs,[53,54] and individual and marital therapy.[22,55,56,57] Now that more than one-quarter of the student population is female, and a substantial number of students are from minority populations, the special issues of these groups must be addressed, including requests for women and minority group therapists to be available.[22]

A real need exists for contemporary studies on the kinds and extent of psychological impairment in the medical student, especially with the change in composition of classes. The data available do not support the assertion that medical students have a high incidence of severe psychopathology. As a group they appear remarkably well selected to complete their studies. They do, however, experience considerable stress for which they should be encouraged to seek help when needed. They need faculty or others who are available and alert to their needs, beyond the demands of the curriculum. The early development of an attitude of responsibility for one's own emotional as well as medical health may succeed in reducing the later prevalence of the impaired physician.

There is an emotional toll even if it is not demonstrated in attrition rates or poor work performance. Reports describing medical student cynicism or disillusionment reveal an unfortunate consequence of a training program that can erode the self-esteem of even highly competent individuals.[41,58] The curriculum needs reassessment; experiences which unnecessarily diminish the student's feeling of competence should be restructured. Most students can adjust more effectively to medical school with support groups, student peer counseling, a responsive faculty and administration, and confidential mental health services.

Some cases illustrate adaptive difficulties of students and a variety of interventions of psychiatrists available to the students.

Case 1

Ann B. had her first contact with Dr. N. in a second-year discussion group for male and female students. Ann was the only minority student in the group, and she had come from another part of the country.

In the group she talked of her isolation, loneliness, and feelings of alienation, but she rarely shared more of her personal thoughts or history. Although initially the other group members found her style of interaction somewhat abrasive, they began to be increasingly more warm and supportive as she spoke more openly. As the group evolved, the students were able to help each other solve concrete problems and also to share anxieties about their current and future roles. They talked about their feelings of inadequacy, their fears about making mistakes, and their concerns about their relationships with friends, lovers, spouses, and parents.

On one occasion Ann called Dr. N. and requested an individual meeting. She stated that she needed to talk about something she couldn't share with the group. She began the meeting with a description of a "put-down" by an instructor who, she felt, saw her as "dumb" because she was a minority student. She quickly shifted to personal issues: her father, she revealed, was a chronic alcoholic who had abandoned the family shortly after she started medical school. Her mother was depressed and very recently had had a coronary so that she could not support the two younger children. Ann wondered whether she should leave school to help the family. Her mother had insisted that she stay at school, but Ann felt guilty.

After two meetings, with Dr. N.'s support she decided to mobilize other family members to help and to remain in school. She did tell the group members this, and in subsequent meetings she let them support her more often.

Formal group meetings ended after one year, but all the members remained in close contact with each other and with Dr. N. They sought each other out during difficult times and saw each other as resources. When Ann's boyfriend left her, she turned to one of the other group members, a man who had had a similar experience. On one occasion during her pediatrics rotation she called Dr. N. to ask how to obtain help for another student whom she felt was depressed. She was pleased and relieved when Dr. N. praised her for her sensitivity and for having taken responsibility for a seriously ill classmate.

Ann disappeared into a hectic round of clerkships. She worked hard, did very well, and occasionally stopped by to see Dr. N. During her fourth year, after internship matching, Ann called again in a crisis. She was disappointed that she had not matched in the program she really wanted, and she was going to a city where she knew nobody. She was frightened and anxious, ·more about her ability to make new relationships than about her ability to function as a physician. She also wanted the name of a therapist, stating that she had to open her "Pandora's Box" sometime. She said that she had learned that there were some things that "one couldn't handle alone." Thanking Dr. N. for being so "important to me" and "helping me bail out," she talked about her need to see "how a woman could do it and survive." She came back just before graduation to tell Dr. N. that she had found an apartment "without cockroaches," because she felt for the first time that she needed to "be better to myself."

This description of the relationship between Ann B. and Dr. N. illustrates several of the issues involved in planning for meeting the complex needs of a diverse group of medical students. Most important is that Ann came to medical school with some special issues related to being a woman, a minority student, and moving into a different cultural context with preexisting, severe family problems preoccupying her. During the course of her education there were additional burdens and stresses, many of which are part of the lives of all students.

As a minority woman in that particular school she had few peers. Furthermore, she moved from a small, less competitive school in a familiar geographical area, with friends and family available, to an alien environment where the demands were high and there were few resources for support. Her ability to cope under pressure was admirable. She could do what successful medical students and physicians learn early—to separate her personal life from her work and to perform to meet expectations.

She made good use of the group. She assessed her own limits and its usefulness to her, and she protected herself in a way which was both characteristic and adaptive, based on her past experience in similar situations. When the stress seemed too great to bear, she was able to find resources, first Dr. N. and gradually others.

Ann could not be described as ill, yet she needed and used services which facilitated optimal personal growth and progress through medical school. It is difficult to know what would have happened had those resources not been available. We do know, however, that students do use resources when they are available.

The task with a student like Ann is to facilitate adaptation, by helping her use her own strengths, and to reinforce her ability to be an active participant in the process. She reinforces the view that when self-esteem is supported and students can achieve a level of mastery, they can better acknowledge the need for help and feel they deserve it. In this situation the combination of the group and a few counseling sessions enabled Ann to cope despite enormous stress. Dr. N. was in part a therapist, in part a counselor and role model, and clearly a friend.

Case 2

Stephen B. was a third-year student on his psychiatry clerkship when he learned that his parents were divorcing after 25 years of marriage. While they had a somewhat tumultuous relationship, Stephen had become sanguine about their stability together. Angry, hurt and sad, he found himself unable to function with his patients. He was distracted and could not listen. He frequently took sides, especially when he saw patients with marital or family problems. As his objectivity and effectiveness decreased, he withdrew to the library or the on-call room where he slept and did not answer his call.

The chief resident informed Dr. N. of the circumstances. He was concerned that Stephen was becoming increasingly more depressed. Furthermore, it did not seem that Stephen could earn a passing grade in psychiatry because of is poor performance. Dr. N. saw Stephen and raised these concerns with him. Stephen was initially defensive, but as they talkd he became more open about his distress. He told Dr. N. that he was scheduled to take his medical clerkship the following month and that he was very worried about performing adequately if he didn't feel better. Dr. N. suggested that he take a few days off, to consider a schedule rearrangement so that he would not feel pressured to perform at a time when he was preoccupied with other issues. Initially he rejected this idea, saying that it would be unfair of him to ask others to cover his patients. After a while, he agreed. He was relieved, but he told Dr. N. that he was afraid that it would "look bad on his record" if he made any changes. Dr. N. was able to reassure him.

Stephen went home for a few days and returned feeling that he could continue the clerkship. He did finish satisfactorily, and he went on to a series of less pressured electives. During this time he also started therapy, after initially expressing concerns about confidentiality, cost, and time. These issues were worked out by referral to a therapist who was not on the medical school faculty and who had some scheduling flexibility, and by arranging a student loan.

Dr. N. saw Stephen again the next year after the senior play, for which he had been an outstanding musical director. He had done well on his medical clerkship 6 months after it was originally scheduled.

This history illustrates another aspect of a role of the psychiatrist. In this situation, as the course director Dr. N. had academic and administrative responsibility, but as a clinician and teacher she had responsibility for the student's well-being. She was able to be supportive as well as concretely helpful. She recognized the validity of his distress and facilitated a constructive approach without damaging his scholastic performance. He was encouraged to seek help in a way that met his needs and concerns most effectively.

Another important aspect of this situation is the management of a crisis situation. The psychiatrist should maintain the position of a concerned faculty member and advisor rather than that of a therapist, while detecting a significant problem, making a successful referral, and preserving the student's self-esteem.

That Stephen was on the psychiatry clerkship may have increased his vulnerability, since the usual adaptive and defensive mechanisms of intellectualization, isolation, displacement, reaction formation, and denial often do not serve as well as in other clinical settings. The stress can, and in this case did, directly parallel the situation to be confronted in the clerkship. At times students who manage to use their usual defense mechanisms appear to be more disturbed because they remain remote and uninvolved and do not perform as well.

Another important aspect of this case is the academic advisory function in which Dr. N. served. Knowing the curriculum and having some latitude to make use of its inherent flexibility, she could help change the environment, and thus in turn support the student at a time when intensifying the stress might have damaged him.

Combining a rearrangement of schedule with short-term therapy can be an extremely successful approach. When handled well, this combination enables students to recognize their vulnerability and accept it as a normal human phenomenon, not as a sign of weakness or inadequacy. The possible impact on patient care is yet to be evaluated, but it is potentially substantial.

Case 3

Dr. N. first heard about Betty C. only two days after the student's obstetrics and gynecology (OB/GYN) clerkship began. The referring teacher, Dr. A., was unclear about the nature of her trouble, but he felt that someone in the student affairs office, especially a psychiatrist, should be alerted. Dr. A. called Dr. N. because he remembered her from a behavioral science course she taught. As he apologetically described Betty's behavior, it became apparent that she was extremely anxious, inappropriate, and paranoid, and that she had a thought disorder. Dr. N. suggested that Betty come to see her as soon as possible. Since Betty had previously met Dr N. on several informal occasions, she agreed.

In Dr. N.'s office Betty, in a somewhat fragmented way, described her "superb" performance on surgery the previous month. She stated that she got along on almost no sleep, worked all the time, and that everyone loved her. When she started OB/GYN, she felt that she was not well received and that people did not trust her. She was enraged by what she saw as poor patient care and felt that she could certainly do a better job. She interspersed these comments with references to her family and social situation, as if she expected Dr. N. to know the circumstances.

Because of Betty's disorganized thinking and difficulty caring for herself, Dr. N. felt that she needed immediate hospitalization and suggested this promptly. Initially Betty weakly protested, but she quickly jumped at Dr. N.'s offer to walk with her to the student health service where arrangements could be discussed and made. She opposed being admitted to a psychiatric unit, but readily agreed to admission to the student infirmary.

She was treated there initially and then voluntarily transferred to a psychiatric unit where she remained for 2 months. Upon her release she and Dr. N. discussed plans for the rest of the year. It seemed to both of them unwise for her to resume work immediately. She was able to obtain a position as a research assistant for one of the professors with whom she had a positive relationship, and she performed well. The following year she reentered medical school and graduated the following June.

This case raises several challenging issues. One important aspect is the use of the network provided by students and faculty who are aware of which faculty members are available and potentially helpful. Both formal and informal networks are used with students as well as colleagues.

In direct encounters in a work context we often do not recognize problems because we deny them or else attribute certain problems only to "patients." At times students and faculty are uncomfortable because they are reluctant to label or define a specific behavior as indicative of psychopathology, or because they are uncertain about the implications of making such a diagnosis. The problem of the role or responsibility (or both) of the medical scool for its graduates is also an issue which must be addressed in the future. While we cannot predict future behavior, we are also responsible to produce competent and stable physicians.

Case 4

John D. was a third-year student who returned to school upset after the summer. He sought out the psychiatrist who had supervised a reading elective in the previous year. During the summer, for the first time in two years he had seen his sister, who had gone for a junior year abroad. She had become increasingly absorbed in religious rituals. Grandiose in her concepts, she had made increasing demands for recognition and care by her family. They were baffled, sensing that something was wrong, but reluctant to seek help because she continued to function well in school. Furthermore, they considered seeing a psychiatrist to be shameful. John had shared that view until he had contact with Dr. N. in medical school.

In his meeting with Dr. N., he requested diagnostic help and suggestions about how to proceed. Concerned that John's sister showed signs of serious emotional disturbance, Dr. N. helped him plan a way to convey the need for a consultation to his parents. She also gave John the names of several potential consultants. He was immensely relieved to have the unequivocal support of a psychiatrist whom he knew and respected, in taking a position which he felt would initially alienate his parents.

In this case the psychiatrist served as a consultant, a resource to the student and his family and a source of support for a new view of his role in the family. Indirectly she also helped consolidate his understanding of an appropriate means of seeking help.

Case 5

Mary E. came from a conventional family which had directed her away from her interest in science and instead supported her in a career as a writer. After several years of working for a local newspaper, marrying, and having a child, she received an assignment to do medical reporting. This reawakened her interest in science and eventually she decided to apply to medical school. Shortly after entering medical school she was aware of feeling depressed. Confused about the depression, she went to talk to the psychiatrist who had interviewed her for admission and had recently given a lecture to her class.

Her anxiety about making a full work commitment was based on concern that she would be interfering with her husband's career and damaging her youngster. As a child, she herself had experienced maternal absence in the atmosphere of poverty in which they lived. Since adequate substitute care was not available, she had numerous caretakers. Her son was at the same age as she had been when she had had a serious childhood illness and had been left alone. The psychiatrist helped her to clarify the basis of her concerns, to assess the various kinds of child-care arrangements which were available, and to make realistic choices. She also supported her in working out shared responsibilities with her husband.

An excellent student, Mary did extremely well. When internship decisions were being made, Mary came back for another visit. She was tempted to choose an exciting but demanding direction and hesitated, wondering again whether she was short-changing her family. Clarifying the issues with the psychiatrist once more made it easier for her to choose. She experienced less guilt, and she worked out special arrangements which would free her to spend critical hours at home.

The psychiatrist was important not only in the conventional role of unofficial short-term therapist, but also by supporting Mary's considering a conflict-producing choice Dr. N. gave her implicit permission to follow her interests and talents. She then facilitated working out the arrangements which would maximize the realization of her goals and take into account her other commitments and concerns.

It is almost a truism to restate that medical students experience considerable stress in the course of their training. They tend to be survivors, who find ways to cope with these stresses and adapt to the complex demands and expectations of the experience. Some of these adaptations may suit them well in the setting of the medical school, but are less adaptive for the demands of practice and family later on. The psychiatrist who works with medical students can fill a number of roles to help promote more successful resolution of distress and conflict. In addition to the traditional clinical role, the psychiatrist has the opportunity to serve as a teacher, advisor, ombudsman, and friend. The psychiatrist can also be a resource for other faculty and administrators in helping them understand and assess the student's problems and facilitate resolutions. These may include a wide range of alternatives in addition to referral for psychotherapy or counseling. Other options include planning sequences and locations of rotations, leaves, support for alternative programs, and the development of group and other avenues of support and contact between students and with faculty.

REFERENCES

1. Cox D: *Youth into Maturity.* New York, Mental Health Materials Center, 1979.
2. Lief HL: Personality characteristics of medical students, in Coombs RH, Vincent CE (eds): *Psychosocial Aspects of Medical Training.* Springfield, Ill, Charles C. Thomas, 1971.
3. Nadelson C, Notman M: Success and failure: Women as medical school applicants. *J Am Med Wom Assoc* 29:167–172, 1974.
4. Kimball C: Medical education as a humanizing process. *J Med Educ* 48:71–77, 1973.
5. Lief HI, Young K, Spruieli V, et al: A psychodynamic study of medical students and their adaptational problems. *J Med Educ* 35:696–704, 1960.
6. McGuire FL: Psycho-social studies of medical students: A critical review. *J Med Educ* 41:424–445, 1961.
7. Miller LB, Erwin EF: A study of attitudes and anxieties in medical students. *J Med Educ* 34:1089–1092, 1959.
8. Saslow G: Psychiatric problems of medical students. *J Med Educ* 31:27–33, 1956.
9. Simon H: Mortality among medical students, 1947 1967. *J Med Educ* 43:1175–1182, 1968.
10. Thomas CB: What becomes of medical students: The dark side. *Johns Hopkins Med J* 138:185–195, 1976.
11. Adsett C: Psychological health of medical students in relation to medical education process. *J Med Educ* 43:728–734, 1968.
12. Eagel J, Smith B: Stresses of the medical student wife. *J Med Educ* 43:840–845, 1968.
13. Edwards M, Zimet C: Problems and concerns among medical students, 1975. *J Med Educ* 51:619–625, 1976.
14. Ginzberg E: *Life Styles of Educated Women.* New York, Columbia University Press, 1966.
15. Hunter, PC, Schwartzman AE: A clinical view of study difficulties in a group of counselled medical students. *J Med Educ* 36:1295–1301, 1961.
16. Johnson D, Hutchins E: Doctor or dropout. *J Med Educ* 32:1113–1269, 1957.
17. Lucas CJ, Kelvin RP, Ojha AB: The psychological health of the pre-clinical medical students. *Br J Psychiat* 111:473–478, 1965.
18. Mudd JW, Siegel R: Sexuality—the experience and anxieties of medical students. *N Engl J Med* 281:1397–1404, 1969.
19. Notman M, Nadelson C, Bennett M: Achievement conflict in women: Psychotherapeutic considerations. *Psychother and Psychosom* 29:203–213, 1978.
20. Roeske N: The quest for role models by women medical students. *J Med Educ* 52:459–466, 1977.
21. Steppacher RC, Mausner JS: Suicide in male and female physicians. *JAMA* 228:323–328, 1974.
22. Nadelson C, Notman M: Adaptations to stress, in Shapiro E, Lowenstein LM (eds): *Becoming a Physician: Development of Values and Attitudes.* Cambridge, Mass, Ballinger, 1979.
23. Everson RB, Fraumeni JF Jr: Mortality among medical students and young physicians. *J Med Educ* 50:809–811, 1975.
24. Epstein C: Encountering the male establishment: Sex status limits on women's careers in the professions. *Am J Sociol* 15:69, 1975.
25. Thomas RB, Luber SA, Smith JA: A survey of alcohol and drug use in medical students. *Dis Nerv System* 38:41–43, 1977.
26. Mechanick P, Mintz J, Gallagher J, et al: Non-medical drug use among medical students. *Arch Gen Psychiat* 29:48–50, 1973.

27. Lipp MR, Benson SG, Taitor Z: Marijuana use by medical students. Am J Psychiat 128:207–212, 1971.
28. Slaby AE, Lieb J, Schwartz AH: Comparative study of the psychosocial correlates of drug use among medical and law students. J Med Educ 47:717–723, 1972.
29. Nadelson C, Notman M: Medical student stress and adaptation. Presented at Annual APA Meeting, Chicago, May 1979.
30. Etzel SI: Medical education in the United States, 1977–78. JAMA 240:2825, 1978.
31. Defries Z, Grothe L: High academic achievement in psychotic students. Am J Psychiat 135:217–219, 1978.
32. Silver LB, Nadelson C, Joseph EJ, et al: Mental health of medical school applicants: The role of the admissions committee. J Med Educ 54(7):534–538, 1979.
33. Vaillant GC, Sobowale N: Some psychological vulnerabilities of physicians. N Engl J Med 287:372–375, 1972.
34. Vaillant GC, Brighton JR, McArthur C: Physicians' use of mood altering drugs: A 20 year follow-up report. N Engl J Med 282:365–370, 1970.
35. Modlin HC, Montes A: Narcotics addiction in physicians. Am J Psychiat 121:358–365, 1964.
36. Hunter RC, Prince R, Schwartzman AE: Comments on emotional disturbances in a medical undergraduate population. Can Med Assoc J 85:989–992, 1961.
37. Pitts FN Jr, Winokur G, Stewart MA: Psychiatric syndromes, anxiety symptoms, and response to stress in medical students. Am J Psychiat 118:333–340, 1961.
38. Golden JS, Marchionne AM, Silver RJ: Fifty medical students: A comparision with "normals." J Med Educ 42-146–152, 1967.
39. Schlageter CW, Rosenthal J: What are "normal" medical students like? J Med Educ 37-19–27, 1962.
40. Keniston K: The medical student. Yale J Biol Med 39:346–356, 1967.
41. Schwartz AH, Swartzburg M, Lieb J. et al: Medical school and the process of disillusionment. J Med Educ 12:182–185, 1978.
42. Coburn D, Jovacas A: Perceived sources of stress among first year medical students. J Med Educ 50:589–595, 1975.
43. Reifler CB, Babineau R: Student mental health services and departments of psychiatry. Am J Psychiat 133:967–969, 1976.
44. Reifler CB: Medical student mental health services. Paper presented at the Annual Meeting of the Association of American Medical Colleges, Washington, DC, Nov. 1978.
45. Bojar S: Psychiatric problems of medical students, in Blaine G, McArthur C (eds): Emotional Problems of the Student, 2d ed.
46. Nelson L: Special problems of graduate students in the school of arts and sciences, in Blaine G, McArthur C (eds): Emotional Problems of the Student, 2d ed. New York, Appleton-Century-Crofts, 1971.
47. Babcock HH: Special problems encountered at the graduate school of business administration, in Blaine G, McArthur C (eds): Emotional Problems of the Student, 2d ed. New York, Appleton-Century-Crofts, 1971.
48. Buckley-Sharp MD: Student breakdown. J of the Royal Society of Med 71:150–151, 1978.
49. Blackwell B: Medical education; Old stresses and new directors. The Pharos, pp. 26–30, January 1977.
50. Rosenberg PP: Students' perceptions and concerns during their first year in medical school. J Med Educ 46:211–218, 1971.
51. Preven D: Unpublished data. 1979.

52. Dashef SS, Espey WM, Lazarus JA: Time limited sensitivity groups for medical students. *Am J Psychiatry* 31:287–292, 1974.
53. Bishop FE, Provenzo EF, Robinson F: A special program for counselling medical students. *J Med Educ* 53:996–997, 1978.
54. Spiro JH, Roenneburg M, Maly BJ: Teaching doctors to treat doctors: Medical peer review. *J Med Educ* 53:997, 1978.
55. Perlow A, Mullins S: Marital satisfaction as perceived by the medical student's spouse. *J Med Educ* 51:726–734, 1976.
56. Porter K, Zeigler P, Charles E, et al: A couples group for medical students. *J Med Educ* 51:418–419, 1976.
57. Robinson DO: Medical student spouse syndrome: Grief reaction to the clinical years. *Am J Psychiatry* 135(8):972–974, 1978.
58. Eron LD: The effect of medical education on attitudes. *J Med Educ* 30:559–566, 1955.

III

Prevention and Treatment of the Impaired Physician

8

Family Therapy for the Impaired Physician

IRA D. GLICK

A colleague told me the following vignette: A 30-year-old, married surgeon with two children came for psychiatric help because of trouble concentrating during operations. He had married during medical school. The early part of the marriage had never stabilized; he and his wife had had frequent disagreements which were never resolved. He had noted an increasing use of alcohol and drugs and had sought psychotherapy. Two days before his most recent appointment for psychotherapy, he performed his usual preoperative routine, saw his patient, whom he had taken care of for many years, and did his operation. Upon leaving the hospital, he realized that he had repeated on that patient the same surgical procedure that he had done two weeks earlier instead of the procedure he had intended to do. He realized that the operation had followed a particularly upsetting argument that he had had with his wife the night before.

WHAT IS THE PROBLEM?

Just as emotional problems affect physicians, so too are they prevalent among their spouses and children. In such families there are well-documented difficulties: inadequate communication, incomplete parental task fulfillment, frustrated dependency needs of spouses, the absence of the physician from the household, and all too often, the lack of a personally meaningful life for the spouse.

IRA D. GLICK • Department of Psychiatry, Cornell University Medical College, New York Hospital–Cornell Medical Center, New York, New York

THE FAMILY MODEL

The family model for understanding how these problems develop suggests, in part, that the impaired physician and the rest of the family are involved in repetitive dysfunctional patterns that lead to psychological symptoms in the physician and often other family members. Until the last 10 years, in the absence of family techniques treatment for the impaired physician was difficult and frequently ineffective. Families were seldom involved in the treatment.[1] My data from treatment of male physicians suggest that family treatment in some cases is an effective intervention in reducing morbidity and increasing function, not only for the identified patient-physicians, but also for their families.*

Family therapy can be considered as any psychosocial intervention using a conceptual framework with primary emphasis on the family system and which, in its therapeutic strategies, aims at affecting the entire family structure. Thus any psychotherapeutic approach that attempts to understand or to intervene in an organically viewed family system might fittingly be called "family therapy." This broad definition allows many differing points of view, both in theory and in therapy, to be placed under one heading.

In many families the members may be "selected" as "symptom bearers." Such individuals will then be described in a variety of ways that will amount to their being labeled "bad," "sick," "stupid," or "crazy." Depending on what sort of label such individuals carry, together with their families, they may be treated in any one of several types of helping facilities: psychiatric, correctional, or medical.

On the other hand there may not always be an *identified patient.* Occasionally a marital or family unit presents itself as being in trouble without singling out any one member. A couple may realize that their marriage is in trouble and that their problems stem from their interaction with each other, not from either partner individually.

There is a continuum between the intrapsychic system, the interactional family system, and the sociocultural system. Different conceptual frameworks apply to each of these systems. A therapist may choose to emphasize any of the points on this continuum, but the family therapist is especially sensitive to and trained in aspects specific to the family system, both to its individual characteristics and to the larger social matrix.

---

* At this writing, I regret that I have too few cases to report in which the impaired physician is a woman. Given current concern for problems of women physicians, they are a group of special interest.

Psychiatric evaluation in such instances focuses not only on the individual but also on the family system. In the case of an impaired physician spouse, such evaluation is crucial in identifying pathology that may cause symptoms in other members of the family. For that reason family therapy is often recommended in situations in which there is severe and chronic marital dissatisfaction, with or without sexual problems, or in which a child or adolescent is the identified problem. Family or marital therapy is utilized when it appears that the identified patient's symptoms are the manifestation of a disturbed family. For example, the impaired physician's spouse presents as the identified patient. Evaluation might suggest that the spouse is the "symptom bearer" for a disturbed family unit or a disturbed physician husband.

In another book I suggest three basic strategies of family therapy:

1. Those that facilitate communication of thoughts and feelings
2. Those that shift disturbed, inflexible roles and coalitions, and
3. Those that aid family role-assumption, education, and demythologizing[2]

These strategies cut across the three usual approaches to the family model:

1. With the insight-awareness approach, observation, clarification, and interpretations are used to foster understanding and, presumably, change.
2. In the structural-behavioral approach, manipulations are devised to alter family structures and conduct.
3. In the experiential approach, emotional experience is designed to change the way family members see and, presumably, react to one another.[2]

WHAT ARE THE CAUSES OF THE PROBLEM?

The physician tends to engage in "selective recruitment when seeking a marriage partner, in the aim of finding someone who will fit in with the single-mindedness of the doctor's lifestyle."[3] For the spouse who sees the physician as a "good catch," this usually means the trade-off of postponing her career. The marital coalition then delays working out the establishment phase of the relationship, a stage in which issues such as sexual satisfaction and role allocation are usually resolved.

The homeostatic balance among demands, responsibilities, and rewards in the impaired physician's family is often delicately maintained. Communication decreases as the physician's work keeps him away from home. Increasingly involved professionally, the physician is no longer available to help the spouse with family tasks, and he gives less attention to her. Over time the spouse feels neglected and acutely aware of the lack of a personally meaningful life. Her narcissistic image changes and she often begins to react differently. She may become angry or withdrawn, or cope by attempting to carve out an identity based on her own, rather than the spouse's ego. This may result in conflict between husband and wife which may cause the physician to have difficulties in his work or to develop symptoms which bring him to psychiatric treatment. The common elements in treatment are how the time taken by the physician's work competes with his involvement at home and how the spouse feels "one-down" as a losing, and boring, competitor.[4]

CASE MATERIAL

I will present short case vignettes both for reasons of confidentiality and because this is a preliminary, uncontrolled report. The focus is on family evaluation and outcome, rather than on process, content, symptoms, or individual psychodynamics, as these have been well described.[5,6,7] Here I will outline situations in which family therapy is useful, compared to other types of psychotherapies, using the data from 10 consecutive physician family referrals.

Case 1

This couple, in their 40s, came to treatment when they felt unable to control their six children, ages 2 to13. One precipitant was that the wife's back problem had worsened and therefore she could not run the household as before; her nephrologist husband had withdrawn from the family. The oldest child, a 13-year-old daughter, had taken over much of the household and parenting responsibilities. The consequences were disastrous, ranging from fights with her 11-year-old sister, rebellion by the four younger siblings, despair and depression in the mother, and further withdrawal by the father. History revealed that both spouses had functioned fairly well before and in the early years of their marriage. Neither was particularly psychologically minded. Treatment suggested was a combination of family therapy and marital therapy, with an emphasis on the former in the beginning part of treatment and the latter in subsequent stages. Treatment goals included: increasing family commu-

Table I. Treatment Outcome for the Impaired Physician and Family[a]

Case	Treatment prescribed	Treatment received and results	Therapist's global rating of treatment outcome								
			For physician			For spouse			For relationship/ marriage/family		
			Imp	Un	Worse	Imp	Un	Worse	Imp	Un	Worse
1	Marital and family therapy	Relationship and family improved	+2			+1			+2		
2	Drug plus family therapy	Spouse refused drug treatment, physician then separated	+2				0				*
3	Marital therapy	Marriage improved	+2			+1			+1		
4	Marital therapy	Relationship improved	+2			+1			+2		
5	Marital and concurrent individual therapy	Couple decided to separate, then reconciled and relationship improved		0		+1			+1		
6	Marital plus drug therapy	Relationship improved	+2			+2			+1		
7	Concurrent individual plus marital therapy	Marital therapy refused by spouse, physician then separated	+2				0				−1*
8	Individual plus marital therapy	Marital therapy refused by spouse, spouse chose concurrent individual therapy, marriage improved, spouse requested marital therapy	+2			+1			+2		
9	Individual therapy plus couple therapy	Relationship improved	+2			+2			+2		
10	Marital therapy	Treatment refused by spouse, relationship unchanged		0		+1				0	

[a] Global rating from −1 to −3 (very much worse), 0 (the same), and +1 to +3 (very much improved). * = Relationship terminated; Imp = Improved; Un = Unimproved.

nication, helping the physician to function as husband and father, encouraging his wife to relinquish some control to him, assisting the children to accept the changes in roles, and supporting the 13-year-old to yield some power over her siblings.

Treatment initially focused on the lack of communication between husband and wife. For the spouse to get her husband's help with the children, she had to become "hysterical." He would withdraw, saying that there was really no problem and that his wife was just a chronic complainer. The older children then filled the power vacuum. The younger children engaged in a variety of attention-seeking behavior such as breaking things, screaming, or holding their breaths until cyanotic. The presence of the wife in the therapeutic sessions forced the physician husband to face the frustration he felt in having to deal with so many offspring (the choice of having the children was his wife's). It also forced him to face, and cope with, problems he was having with his partners in his practice. The husband realigned his roles, taking over some of the parenting and spending fewer hours at work.

After one year of family treatment with eight family members, and marital treatment, the physician improved markedly. He functioned better in his practice and as a husband and father. His wife improved as well; she had moderate relief from her back pain, when she could seek appropriate medical attention and did not have to carry the burden of the house "on her back." The older children were able to stop being parent substitutes, and the younger children did better in school and were better able to accept limits.

Case 2

This physician, in his 50s, came to treatment after a five-year course of psychoanalysis for his wife failed to improve her paranoid and delusional symptoms. Evaluation revealed that she had chronic schizophrenia, had refused medication, and was still delusional. The husband and the children felt that they could not live with her illness anymore. His work was impaired.

The evaluation focused on the state of the marriage, whereas previous treatment had attended to the intrapsychic conflicts of the wife. Now there was virtually no relationship between the couple, in part because the wife was quite psychotic, manifesting a thought disorder including blocking and loose associations. She was unable to communicate with her husband or their children. The treatment suggested was medication for the wife as an individual and family therapy.

The wife refused medications. Following two family therapy sessions, the husband decided to separate from her. The outcome, a year later, was that husband and children were more functional but the wife was unchanged.

Case 3

This couple, in their early 30s, came to treatment because the wife was considering having an affair. Evaluation showed that although they had known each other since their teens, the wife had always felt subordinate in the relationship. She had sacrificed her career. She felt that he placed his professional work as a psychiatrist ahead of her and treated her like "one of the boys." She suggested marital therapy as a step before separating. Marital therapy was recommended.

Treatment in this case focused on roles. This couple had functioned in a typical one-up/one-down model, with the spouse feeling demeaned and withdrawing from her husband. She fantasized initiating an affair; when she told her husband about it, he was patronizing and aloof. The therapy forced him to evaluate the effect of his behavior on his wife. He had to increase his communication, which earlier had been mostly perfunctory and focused on her meeting his needs. Follow-up 6 months later revealed that "they were closer than ever before," and they were planning to have a child.

After one year of weekly sessions there was marked improvement in the marriage and in each of them individually.

Case 4

This couple, in their 40s, came to treatment as the wife's career as an artist was developing. Each had been married once before. The ostensible reason for therapy was that the spouse, who was in individual psychotherapy, complained constantly about her husband. Treatment suggested was marital therapy.

Six weeks of weekly marital therapy focused on communication, changes in role, and decreasing the sexual distance between the couple. In typical fashion, the physician husband tended to demean his spouse as "the sick one," while she felt that he was withdrawn and cold. He believed that he was not being appreciated for the amount of money he was bringing in and for how hard he was working. Therapy focused on altering roles and increasing communication, and gradually fostering intimacy through a series of prescribed exercises. The couple was able to work on tasks, including developing a budget.

Both individuals and their relationship improved. Interestingly, the wife found the therapy more difficult than did her husband because it changed her image of him—for the better!

Case 5

This couple, in their 20s, came to treatment following the wife's discovery of her surgeon husband's affair. Evaluation revealed that he had been the only child of indulgent parents. The spouse was from a family in which the father had done a "lot of running around." She had two older sisters and had to "share parents' love." She felt she "was not needed." Treatment suggested was individual therapy, plus marital therapy on alternate weeks.

The treatment focused on both working out some of the core individual conflicts which complicated the marital relationship. The physician husband felt that he was too busy at work to take care of the house, preferring, when home, to sit in front of the television set to "leave the hospital behind." Although their sexual activity was adequate, it had markedly decreased in frequency and in satisfaction from the onset of marriage. The marital therapy made the physician husband face his unspoken need for his wife to take care of him. In individual therapy he had to attend to his strong and unresolved dependency needs.

After 6 months the couple decided to separate, realizing that they were unable to accommodate each other's fantasies and needs. She wanted a strong man and he was dependent; he wanted to be taken care of and she did not want to do that. The physician husband was unchanged, but the spouse felt markedly better. They then reconciled and improved, as therapy helped them shape the relationship to the realities of each of their personalities.

Case 6

This couple, in their 40s, asked for treatment following the "failure of each of their psychoanalyses to resolve marital discord." The physician husband consistently treated his wife as a patient, and in fact had been prescribing antidepressant medication for her. Evaluation indicated that both partners had a major depressive disorder. Treatment suggested was marital therapy and antidepressant medication for both.

Two months after beginning medication there was moderate improvement for each individual and for the relationship. They began to stop blaming each other for a lack of their enjoyment of life and started to communicate. The phyician husband had spent long hours in his practice and neglected his role as father and husband. Communication had been difficult because of mutual blame when one or the other felt "low."

Follow-up 6 months later revealed that the wife had discontinued medication because she gained weight. The cycle of mutual blaming followed, withdrawal of the physician husband continued, and the couple decided to separate.

Case 7

This 30-year-old radiologist came to therapy because of an acute crisis with his wife of 2 years. Over the past 7 months she had been "coming and going," and his anxious rumination was interfering with his work. His 25-year-old wife had a long history of short-lived relationships which she initiated and then broke off. Marital treatment was recommended. When the wife refused, the physician began individual treatment. He then separated from her, but continued in individual therapy, with his wife coming for two marital sessions. Subsequent follow-up indicated that he felt markedly improved and functioned significantly better at his job. They divorced, and he eventually formed another relationship. His former wife continued to have a chaotic course in and out of a number of tumultuous relationships.

Case 8

This couple, in their 40s, came to treatment when the spouse wanted a divorce from her internist husband. Evaluation of the situation revealed that she had long resented his frequent absences from home and his professional demands. She correctly perceived that he was insensitive to her needs. She had recently initiated an affair with another physician and was now threatening divorce. Marital therapy was recommended. The wife refused, choosing individual psychotherapy. Individual treatment was then also prescribed for the internist. Following 4 months of treatment the marriage improved, as did both individuals. At this point the spouse requested marital therapy. All improved: the spouse, the physician, and their relationship.

This case suggests that the spouse forced her physician husband to face chronic problems such as his lack of communication, his insensitivity to her needs, and his inability to fulfill the role demands of a relationship. Positive changes in both members resulted.

Case 9

This 28-year-old pediatrician came for individual therapy after a divorce and a new engagement, which he described as mildly conflicted. He believed the blame was his, since both relationships had similar problems. Individual therapy was suggested for the physician, followed in 3 months by couple therapy.

His fiancée was able to confront the physician with his fears of intimacy, with his needs to be one-up in the relationship and to discourage her career. Two months of couple therapy, focusing on communication, role change, and issues around intimacy, resulted in improvement in the couple. Six-month followup revealed that both had maintained the gains.

Case 10

This psychiatrist and his spouse, both in their 60s, came to therapy as their children were leaving home. Evaluation indicated that the physician husband had a chronic schizophrenic disorder and was barely functional. Over the past 5 years the wife had considered leaving the marriage. The treatment suggested was marital therapy. She refused. There was no change in either the spouse or the physician husband, although the wife reported that the relationship was better, as somehow the consultation had "helped."

In this case, using the marital model resulted in forcing the issue of whether or not to separate. Although at the time of the evaluation the spouse decided to stay, 2 years later she separated from her husband.

WHAT ARE THE MARITAL AND FAMILY THERAPY INTERVENTIONS NEEDED?

It is obvious from the foregoing cases that the choice of treatment varies with the needs of the family. The choice can be:

1. Individual psychotherapy for the identified patient
2. Individual psychotherapy for both physician and spouse
3. Marital therapy or family therapy alone, or in combination with 1 or 2

Individual therapy for impaired physicians has reportedly been difficult because of their characteristic narcissism, and use of reaction formation and of denial. Often these problems are unworkable and treatment is ineffective. Concurrent individual therapy for physician and spouse may be indicated when the relationship is too emotionally charged for the couple to be seen together. The approach suggested by this experience and in another report of two cases[8] is marital or family therapy, based on the rationale that family structure and function must change in order for the identified physician-patient to change.

Goals of marital or family treatment rest on the following principles. First, communication must increase, e.g., by establishing daily time for this between the physician, his spouse, and other family members. Second, the roles for the impaired physician and his spouse must change. Most commonly he abrogates his role as a husband or parent or both; he must assume more household and parental responsibilities. The spouse must be aided by the therapist in assuming her new identity. Third, the children must be helped to feel comfortable in accepting the new roles of their parents. Case 1 illustrates this problem most pointedly, for the therapist had to assist the children to accept control from the parents rather than from the 13-year-old who had been in charge of the family.

Finally, what are the results for the impaired physician? These data illustrate that overall results are good. The reasons are currently speculative. I suggest that the presence of the spouse forces the impaired physician to confront problems rather than denying them, and offers an alternative view to his injured narcissism. Further, she serves as a control to prevent the impaired physician's self-destructive behavior and motivates change by threatening separation if "things don't improve." At the very least such an approach increases communication between the couple.

Controlled studies are needed to develop a basis for predicting which type of treatment is best for which patient, spouse, and family. Data are also needed on impaired female physicians and their families. The family treatment offers a viable alternative to the individual approach. In a unique way, involving the family cuts through the impaired physician's denial. It can lead to role examination and aid treatment compliance. Controlled outcome studies comparing family therapy to other therapies are needed to test this and other assumptions.

REFERENCES

1. Waring EM: Medical professionals with emotional illness: A controlled study of the hazards of being a "special patient." *Psychiat J Univ Ottowa* 4:161–164, 1977.
2. Glick ID, Kessler DR: *Marital and Family Therapy*, 2d ed. New York, Grune & Straton, 1980, pp 6, 126, 128.
3. Deckert G: Personal communication, 1979.

4. Borus J: Personal communication, 1980.
5. Waring EM: Psychiatric illness in physicians: A review. *Compr Psychiat* 15:519–530, 1974.
6. Scheiber SC: Emotional problems of physicians: I. Nature and extent of problems *Ariz Med* 34:323–325, 1977.
7. Scheiber SC: Emotional problems of physicians: II. Current approaches to the problem. *Ariz Med* 35:336–337, 1978.
8. Krell R, Miles JE: Marital therapy of couples in which the husband is a physician. *Am J Psychotherapy* 30-267–275, 1976.

9

Psychotherapeutic Issues in Psychiatric Treatment of Physicians with Alcohol and Drug Abuse Problems

THOMAS G. WEBSTER

More psychiatrists are now apt to see physicians with alcohol and drug-abuse problems. Such physicians are more apt to appear at earlier stages, in milder degree, and on an outpatient basis. Mobilization of organized medicine's attention to problems of the impaired physician is already yielding results, yet has a long way to go.

Most psychiatric studies reported in the literature are on advanced cases of hospitalized physicians, often those identified to medical societies or state licensure boards. The magnitude of the problem is large. Problems of motivation for psychiatric treatment are common. Attitudes of the physician's medical colleagues may help or hinder referral for psychiatric treatment. Psychiatrists may also have stereotyped, stigmatizing, or overly pessimistic attitudes about treatment of persons for substance abuse. Whether from the viewpoint of the physician, his or her colleagues, or the psychiatrist, these prejudices are part of the problem.

Drug-addicted physicians differ from the typical drug abuser in several respects,[1] including economics, education, family, age of onset, choice of drug, socialization with nonabusers, and a greater tendency to use the drug for coping rather than for pleasure. Statewide programs for physicians with alcohol and drug abuse, such as in Georgia, Indiana, California, Virginia, Wisconsin, and New York, have been intensified and they are indicating improved treatment programs and better prognosis than in earlier reports.[2-6] For example, in Georgia during the first 2 years of the

THOMAS G. WEBSTER ● Department of Psychiatry and Behavioral Sciences, and Department of Child Health and Development, George Washington University School of Medicine and Health Sciences, Washington, D.C.

Georgia Disabled Doctor Program, 1975–1977, 20 cases were found who voluntarily suspended practicing medicine, successfully went through treatment and came back to work, without one name being revealed to the state licensing board.[2,7] For each one of these physicians there are presumably even more who have earlier, milder problems of substance abuse as well as those with more serious problems that have not yet been identified or received adequate attention.

The best available estimates are that about 7% of physicians will suffer from alcoholism and 1% from narcotic addiction during their careers.[8,9] For example, this represents about 800 physicians in Georgia, which has roughly 11,500 practicing physicians. Bisell and Jones, in a retrospective study,[8] reported on 98 recovered alcoholic physicians all of whom had been entirely abstinent for at least 1 year. The authors reported that one-third of the physician-patients claimed that their previous psychiatrists did not identify their principal problem as drug or alcohol abuse. Thus these psychiatrists who had previously treated the physician-patients reportedly tended to other aspects of the patient's problems while not focusing on the substance abuse.

For each identified case there are still more with mild forms of drug and alcohol abuse. Many of them may never develop more serious cases of disabling addiction. However, all are in distress, and a few are presumably already seeing psychiatrists privately. All are in double jeopardy. Current mushrooming efforts will better identify such cases and offer them hope by which they will be more apt to seek help voluntarily. More intensive work at the medical student and residency level is also apt to increase future requests for earlier intervention by psychiatrists in substance abuse by practicing physicians. More psychiatrists likely will be called upon to provide treatment in private practice settings.

Psychiatric treatment and psychotherapy issues are somewhat different for different stages or degrees of severity of substance abuse in physicians. For purposes of discussion four stages are listed:

Stage 1. Alcohol or drug abuse is mild or intermittent, often not the chief complaint. Substance abuse may be hidden initially.

Stage 2. Alcohol drug abuse is clearly a prominent problem, even if the doctor is functioning fairly well and minimizing his or her loss of control.

Stage 3. Hospitalization has occurred or is indicated for psychiatric symptoms or impaired behavior with alcoholism and/or drug addiction.

Stage 4. The doctor has deteriorated in his functioning secondary to alcohol or drug addiction. He has "hit bottom." He is more amenable to and shows greater acceptance of confrontation techniques, and is more willing to face the reality of his illness, patient role, dependency, Alcoholics Anonymous, and/or other treatment and rehabilitation modalities.

The above stages are not sharply demarcated. Stage 4, "hit bottom," cannot be fully established except by the subsequent course. An important objective is to establish an effective therapeutic alliance with the patient during Stage 1 or 2 versus Stage 3 or 4. Such an alliance would provide a potential for turnabout and improvement in stages as early as possible. The task of psychotherapy is to provide effective and specific ego support before the physician's reduced self-esteem, personal isolation, and rigid defenses become established and require more crushing external confrontation.

This chapter focuses primarily on psychotherapeutic issues in early intervention, Stage 1 and partly Stage 2. The basic principles apply to all stages. Treatment of Stages 3 and 4 have received more attention in published reports. Changes in the psychodynamics and psychotherapeutic methods with advancing stages will be discussed.

REFERRAL AND ENTRY INTO CONSULTATION OR THERAPY

In early stages referral is apt to be a combination of informal contacts and self-referral. The following are examples: (1) The physician may contact a physician friend, sometimes from out of town, who is either a psychiatrist or psychiatrically oriented and who assists in referral. (2) The physician may be gently confronted by a comment from a physician friend or colleague regarding his not appearing his usual self, then accept referral. (3) The physician may be referred by his or her own internist or family physician as a more formal referral relevant to physical health but with a personal touch. (4) The physician may spontaneously seek out a psychiatrist who was encountered earlier in medical school or residency with whom the physician feels at ease. In most of these circumstances there is a premium on some friendship or a comfortable acquaintance between the psychiatrist and a medical colleague somewhere in the picture. Contributions by psychiatrists to early intervention are heavily dependent on fostering such friendships and professional liaisons.

A premium on privacy also exists. Private offices rather than institutional settings are usually desired. In group-practice settings it is important to provide the physician-patient reasonable anonymity from other patients at the psychiatrist's office. In more advanced cases the tendency of physicians to seek out private facilities, such as the Menninger Clinic or Mayo Clinic, is indicative of the desire for privacy, distance from the local setting, and a reputation for clinical expertise.[10,11] In my own experience with various roles in the referral and treatment process, I am impressed that physician-patients seek high quality of care combined with personal qualities of the psychiatrist with whom they anticipate talking comfortably. Unlike some medical or surgical illnesses which would require specialized tertiary care settings, it is less likely that physicians would seek out research settings for the evaluation and care of early problems with substance abuse.

PERSONAL AND PROFESSIONAL RESPECT

Professional respect is easier to maintain on initial contacts with physician-patients than in some later circumstances, particularly when dealing with alcoholism and drug addiciton. Maintaining both empathy and objectivity in the face of denial, manipulation, frustration, and/or failures in treatment can be difficult. Another side to the problem is something resembling the VIP syndrome. Out of some combination of respect, awe, and timidity, the therapist may lean over backward to avoid being overly intrusive or offending to the physician-patient. Connelly emphasized that "the physician-patient must be thought of first as a person with alcoholism, and second as a physician."[12] Several authors have commented on the reluctance of many physicians to get involved in referral for treatment of physician colleagues with alcoholism or drug abuse.[1-3,5,6,8,12]

Good will is not enough. In consultation or therapy the psychiatrist needs to elicit concrete data from the patient. The treating psychiatrist has to develop genuine respect and warmth for the physician-patient. When the patient appears overly concerned to put his best foot forward, this should not be interpreted simply as defensive. It is symptomatic of a message that must be heard and convincingly reflected in the psychiatrist's reactions and attitudes. Otherwise the problems that are immersed in humiliation are not apt to be brought into the proposed therapeutic solution.

Psychotherapeutic dilemmas include timing and the relative emphasis on tenderness mixed with reminders of hard facts. Clinical judgment is needed to determine when to support the physician's idealism and social consciousness. Also, supporting the realities of his victimization from others, from drugs, and from the patient's own conscience have to be addressed judiciously.

Trust must be built over time based on the way the psychiatrist handles specific critical incidents. Trust is also built by the basic respectful attitudes mentioned above and by making the conditions of therapy explicit. Explicit conditions should include factors of confidentiality and the psychiatirst's contacts with persons other than the physician-patient regarding his case.

The psychotherapeutic alliance is probably the most crucial aspect of early contacts of physician-patients with psychiatrists. Whether the physician is seen for consultation or for treatment of symptoms or for help with "a problem," there is a great premium on identifying and working with the physician's own view and purpose in seeing the psychiatrist. The physican's traditional orientation for requesting diagnostic assessment and expert advice must be heeded, even though such expressed desires can also be deceptive. The physician's need for independent judgment, even competitive views, and the need for maintaining a sense of self-control are apt to be very strong. Many physicians with substance abuse are not especially psychologically minded. They are apt to be persons of action dealing with external variables. The psychiatrist should clearly distinguish in his own mind what is emotional insight and self-awareness and what is intellectual interest. The physician's apparent interest in the psychiatrist's psychodynamic concepts or perception of problems may be seductive and misleading if the physician has not already concretely identified the problem or its components in the physician's own experience and words.

For example, a physician sought my help for symptoms of anxiety with some depression, associated with a major opportunity and decision in his professional life. He had begun self-medication with a tricyclic antidepressant in small doses. He seemed reasonably satisfied with the results. I was concerned with his use of that particular drug. I thought that the anxiety was probably somewhat reinforced and prolonged by the medication. However, I also took note of the small dose and his reported satisfaction. In the absence of clearer evidence of a detrimental effect, I chose to reconcile myself to the fact that at that time the patient saw medication more as part of a self-controlled solution than as part of the problem. At that time I did not comment on his choice of medication.

The physician's major anxiety centered on fear of loss of control in his life-problem situation. I reinforced evidence of his strength and control, based on historical evidence and his responses in the interviews. When, two sessions later, he commented on his desire and intent to taper off the medication, I gently concurred, pointing out the evidence of how well he was managing otherwise. I also indicated that he could be guided by his own observations of the evidence in the future; for example, how well did he maintain his confidence, free of recurrent distress, as he gradually tapered off the drug? His subsequent success in this regard further reinforced his confidence in himself and in me, and thereby reduced his sense of the power of drugs as the key to recovery.

Only later, weeks after he had discontinued the drug, and as part of the termination process, did I raise the issue of drug choice and dosage. He then spontaneously commented that in retrospect he seriously doubted the usefulness of the medication, though at the time he felt he had to do something. This also occurred in the context where he had developed more trust in me and in his ability to use my services helpfully. So the idea of seeking guidance as to medication and seeking psychiatric help more readily were part of the alliance. This orientation came more spontaneously from him than if I had attempted to give him the benefit of all I knew and all he did not know about psychoactive drugs at an earlier stage in therapy.

While there is a definite need and place for confrontation, this must be done carefully within the context of the therapeutic alliance. I tend to err on the cautious side, particularly with physician-patients where the therapist's authority and control are apt to be met with ambivalance if not resistance. Physician patients also struggle with their own authority and control. At later stages, when a greater climate of trust has increased the credibility of the therapist, it is more feasible to confront more actively. As trust builds, the therapeutic alliance is less fragile.

In early interventions the creation of a working relation is paramount. The patient may likely return in time of future self-felt need. Establishing a relationship is a much more crucial early treatment goal than using authoritative advice at the expense of a therapeutic alliance. The same principle applies to an overly ambitious undertaking of psychotherapy during the first sequence of visits. This is true even if the physician agrees to cooperate and intellectually subscribes to treatment in the face of strong passive or active signs that he is resisting. In more advanced stages of alcohol and drug dependency, firm confrontation and external controls take on a much higher priority.

When establishing areas of agreement in the alliance, it is also important to maintain awareness of the limitations and sometimes make these limitations explicit. Limitations may be overlooked or misjudged by overidealization, by unspoken assumptions by patient or therapist, or by verbal agreements which subsequent behavior fails to fulfill. The building of an alliance must occur gradually. The evidence must be clear and convincing to the patient. The therapist may need to point out such evidence and make new areas of agreement quite explicit at times. Consistency in attitude and behavior on the therapist's part are crucial. The therapist should avoid assuming compliance or making verbal agreements that may well be beyond the patient's capacity to fulfill. The subtle versions are more difficult to deal with than the classic "I'll never take another drink, doc."

A particularly important element in therapy, which often involves a dilemma for clinical judgment, is the evolution of the therapeutic alliance in a manner that assists the patient in voluntarily gaining assistance by means of external controls. The external control may be from the therapist, treatment team, family, or organized medical groups. The greater the patient's genuine choice of external control based on his enlightened self-interest, the greater his sense of self-control. He thereby acknowledges his own limitations while at the same time exercising wisdom in caring for himself. This point may need to be emphasized, and is not firmly established until it is manifest in the patient's attitude and behavior. For example, one patient enlisted his wife and me, and on one occasion requested hospitalization when in therapy he came to recognize and accept his own "blind spots" and had experienced concretely the value of the voluntary external controls at home and at work. This is easier said than done. Often an external threat of involuntary control, such as loss of medical practice privileges, is necessary and effective for reinforcing voluntary external controls as a component of the therapeutic alliance. Examples are described in the reports of state medical programs.

DRUG AND ALCOHOL DEPENDENCE

Drug or alcohol dependency is a specific problem that should be addressed somewhat independently for what it is, regardless of associated psychodynamic factors. Again, Bissell and Jones found that recovered alcoholic patients emphasized this as a major complaint about their earlier experiences with psychiatrists.[8] The fact of substance dependency should be established as early as possible within the context of the treatment alliance and treatment goals. This introduces early, even "prematurely" in some cases, the need for agreements as to external controls while the establishment of basic trust and alliance is still at an early tenuous stage. Herein is one of the major dilemmas of therapy, which calls for clinical experience and judgment. It requires more explicit attention than often occurs in the initial stages of psychotherapy.

At first the above statements may sound inconsistent with the case illustration I used earlier regarding the therapeutic alliance. However, that physician-patient was an example of self-medication to reduce the symptoms of an acute situational reaction, not drug dependency. One can easily see the potential for drug dependency in such a case, if untreated. Without psychotherapy that physician could conceivably have had a conditioning reinforcement that self-medication meant self-control in the face of anxiety about loss of control. This could falsely give him the illusion of continuing self-control through continuing self-medication. In many cases of physician drug abuse that process has occurred.

The following is a case illustrating the need for specific attention to substance dependency regardless of associated factors. Another physician consulted me for depressive symptoms, for which she too had tried self-medications with an antidepressant in small doses. She was definitely depressed, both mildly on a chronic basis and more severely on an acute basis in reaction to a serious illness in a close family member. She was not self-referred, and this proved to be consistent with other limitations in her motivation. However, she had accepted the spontaneous advice of a friend and colleague who commented that she appeared depressed and suggested that she see me. Neither was a psychiatrist.

The therapeutic alliance was fostered by my prescribing an antidepressant similar to, although different from, her self-medication. I also prescribed a higher, more consistent, and therapeutic dosage. In doing so, I supported her by clearly indicating that part of her own decision was a step in the right direction. I chose not to mention her errors in dosage. This alliance was increased when her depression gradually lifted.

In regard to psychotherapy, an uneasy therapeutic alliance existed with this physician-patient. However, the alliance was crucial in the long run. Psychotherapy was intellectually acceptable, but she was not very emotionally insightful. She initially accepted weekly psychotherapy on the basis of my authority and advice as a physician, but with ambivalence. She was uncomfortable with "the crutch" nature of seeing me regularly. Yet during each session she readily poured out a list of many reality stresses with which she had to contend. This process continued after the depression lifted, but without the burdensome pessimism that accompanied the depression.

One of the factors that held her in therapy, despite her ambivalence, was her gradual use of therapy for help with specific patients and family members. This particularly applied where emotions were involved and where the physician-patient had received complaints from patients, nurses, or family about her behavior. The alliance was further reinforced by a less conscious dependency and support, as from a friend to an emotionally isolated physician. It is important to note that this physician-patient had many friends and was not socially isolated. Her initial emotional isolation improved significantly with therapy, though a long-standing residual remained. Also, some insight therapy did occur (details are not reported here because the issues were more specific to the individual physician than to the particular issues of substance abuse in the physician-patient).

The next issue in therapy was substance dependency. After several months it became clear that she was dependent on a minimum of two glasses of bourbon in the evenings and again upon awakening in the middle of each night. This behavior had antedated her depressive episode and persisted after the more serious acute depression lifted. This alcohol dependency would not have been broached if she were treated with antidepressants without an effective psychotherapeutic alliance. She would consider the bourbon to be within the realm of moderate drinking, but she was dependent on it and usually took even more on weekends or when sleeplessness indicated. I advised her to increase the antidepressant medication despite feeling less depressed, and I did not stop the antidepressant until she could get through the night regularly without the alcohol. I followed her progress by occasional questions about alcohol use during interviews that dealt mainly with other material. Several weeks after stopping the antidepressant medication the physician-patient had resumed her nighttime drinking on an occasional basis, though not so much nor as regularly as before.

My therapeutic dilemma about termination at this point involved the fact that her alcohol dependency had been broken, even if temporarily, and the patient was relieved of most of her depressive symptoms. The depressive symptoms were what brought her to me, with encouragement from a physician colleague; relief from depressive symptoms was the principal basis for the alliance. The hazards of further use of alcohol to relieve symptoms was not firmly within the functioning therapeutic agreement, nor was the total abstinence. Indeed, the alliance about the drinking had from the beginning been somewhat externally imposed by me despite the patient's gradual cooperation. She had eventually accepted more responsibility for setting future psychotherapy appointments rather than making it seem more like doctor's orders from me. After 1 year of therapy with a gradual decrease in frequency of appointments, a mild temporary recurrence of depressive symptoms augmented her motivation to continue in therapy. This occurred around the anniversary of her first visit and shortly after the departure of her college-age sons who had been home for the Christmas holidays.

After a recovery from this mild recurrence of depressive symptoms, for which no antidepressant medication was necessary, I was prepared to accept termination of therapy at her suggestion. This acceptance on my part was despite a reasonably high likelihood of her return to at least minor alcohol dependency and a continuing but reduced susceptibility to reactive depressive episodes. She was now at least intellectually more aware of the potential hazards of regular use of alcohol; she had reason to associate the therapy with her own success in mastering the many stresses that she had to face; her work and income were steadier; and she associated the therapeutic work with relief of depressive symptoms when they occurred. After 9 months of calling the alcohol issue to her attention with at least temporary success, I felt that to press further without her firm commitment would overly erode the working relationship we had established. I would become too much of a superego figure, which she strongly defended against, and not so much an ego ally, which was the basis of our work together and her experience of success. By now terminating at her suggestion, which I had resisted earlier, I felt she was more apt to return to see me when in future need.

INVOLVEMENT OF THE FAMILY

Involvement of the family is strongly indicated but also requires clinical judgment and specificity in assessment and management. The well-being of family members as individuals may sometimes merit specific attention that is not in all dimensions consistent with their role as a support system for the physician. Work with families in different stages should be distinguished from those periods in Stages 3 and 4 when it is important for all to rally in support of the physician's recovery. Groups such as Al-Anon as an adjunct to Alcoholics Anonymous provide for needs of family members as well as for the physician-patient.[13]

Another case example involved a young physician-patient whose wife was the principal and virtually only source of emotional support. My concerns in this case, in addition to help with an acute transient situational reaction, had to do with future years when the physician would have increased practice responsibilities and the wife would have greater family responsibilities. At such a future time his sole reliance on the spouse for support would run the risk of deterioration of their successful but isolated two-way support system. The physician's contact with a psychiatrist for brief symptoms was thus used for a secondary preventive function. I made it a point to manage the brief contact with this physician-patient and with his wife in a manner to lower the threshold for their reaching out early in the event of some future crisis or marital distress.

Treatment in the Advancing Stages

In the more advanced stages of alcoholism and drug addiction, Stages 3 and 4, the basic objectives and issues of psychotherapy remain the same. However, significant modifications occur by virtue of the new elements in the picture. These new elements include: (1) more serious symptoms and psychopathology; (2) a shifting of ego defenses and superego forces whether in illness or recovery, usually involving a more intensive regression; (3) greater loss of privacy; (4) more external controls, such as the hospital, expanded treatment team, medical society, licensure board, courts, AA, or similar groups; (5) more prominent physical, physiological, and pharmacological factors; and (6) new and usually expanded interpersonal contacts and a more diversified support system. In all stages, with or without contacts with a psychiatrist, state medical society programs and other new resources are more commonly coming into play.[14-19] Outreach programs, such as the case-finding methods of the Georgia plan or the Physicians Confidential Hotline of the California Medical Society, bring external resources and often external controls into the picture at an earlier than usual stage of the physician's substance dependency.[2,4] Advanced stages of illness and more extreme measures may thus be averted. Voluntary individual psychotherapy may often be enhanced in such cases, despite added complications compared to more totally voluntary treatment.

To oversimplify for the sake of clarity, superego functions become more prominent in advancing stages, both in illness and in recovery. Differences in character structure are presumably involved, but the nature of the illness and the cumulative toll on the people involved are also powerful reinforcers. From the psychotherapeutic standpoint some alternative ego functions may be surrendered in the process, at least temporarily and sometimes for years or a lifetime. The individual psychotherapist, generally committed to a nonjudgmental reality orientation, including confrontation but not moralizing, may have a lesser or modified task in the treatment of these advanced stages. By more prominent superego functions, I loosely refer to the direct manifestations such as embarrassment, humiliation, shame, loss of self-esteem, social isolation, depression, helplessness, and hopelessness. Defenses against these influences may be even more prominent, such as denial of illness and failures, projection of blame on externals, superindependence, and even grandiosity.

While ego and superego functions are always at work in varying proportions, the solution based on superego functions that comes with "hitting bottom" resembles a conversion after going to the sinner's bench as much as recovery from illness. This rebirth or "second genesis" includes a new self-image as a recovered alcoholic or ex-addict. A counter-compulsion, or total abstinence, may be necessary in many cases to replace the compulsion to drink or to self-medicate. Ego functions become remobilized around this new identity. The therapists in such a process tend to involve groups which share the superego and then ego functions. Inspiration, idealization, moral judgment, and exhortation are much more familiar in such groups than in usual individual psychotherapy. Interdependency, common identity, and structured rules are also crucial factors. Recovered alcoholic or formerly addicted physicians are especially valuable assets, such as described in the Georgia program. The same can be said of the family when they have been participants in the recovery process.

Individual and group therapies may be mutually supportive as required. Individual psychotherapists and one-to-one relations often do not have a prominent place in such treatment and rehabilitation processes. The therapist supports the group methods and the patient's use of them, sometimes with a privately held aversion to some features. However, individual patients have different patterns and the role of individual therapy varies widely during and after such group processes in Stages 3 and 4.

The main point is for the psychiatrist to have an awareness of the complexity of the psychodynamics in the individual patient and the relative usefulness and limitations of individual, group, and family therapy. An increasing orientation to the reality of physiological and chemical dependency, including genetic factors, has helped increase a nonjudgmental ego orientation on the part of patients and those who work with them. However, this concept can also be used by the patient as a rationalization or excuse to the punishing superego. Superego function, healthy and otherwise, will likely always have a prominent place in the illness and recovery of a significant number of patients.

Hospitalization has a key role not only in the management of detoxification and medical problems, but in establishing firm working relationships with an eye to the rehabilitation period ahead.[13] Unfortunately, some inpatient units tend to limit treatment to the immediate symptoms and their management during brief hospitalizations. This orientation tends to neglect continuity of care and the opportunity to establish future psychotherapy and rehabilitation on a more solid base. The problem is accentuated when the hospital is isolated geographically from the patient's home.

In treatment during all stages of severity, the role of the psychiatrist can be particularly significant in integrating physical and pharmacological aspects of the treatment with psychiatric assessment and psychotherapy. These functions may also be split in the treatment team, particularly during Stages 3 and 4, often with greater reliance on superego mechanisms via nonmedical counselors or therapists or by nonpsychiatric physicians. Behavior modification is useful for specific behavioral symptoms that bring many secondary complications. All such treatment components should be integrated into a comprehensive treatment approach in which the total patient is central, not fragmented.

The psychiatrist, doing individual psychotherapy in a private office setting, has a significant responsibility for overall case management. Work with the family and collaboration with professional colleagues are essential in Stages 2, 3, and 4, regardless of the division of labor. Inherent to this function are several psychotherapeutic issues requiring skilled clinical judgment. Examples include administrative-therapist splits, drug management-psychotherapy combinations, orientation to external controls, relative degrees of privacy and confidentiality, questions of communications with the medical society and licensure board, and the psychiatrist's relation to support groups such as AA, recovered physician counselors, and employers. Each of these dilemmas has a counterpart within the patient's mind and in the psychotherapeutic relation.

Finally, the psychiatrist, when called upon, provides another important factor at any stage in the treatment—hope. Fortunately, this may now be based on cumulative demonstrated evidence, which in the end may be the strongest inspiration. The therapist, however, should maintain a realistic orientation and not desert the patient's grief, pain, and other distress, for which there is also abundant evidence.

In summary, stereotypes of alcoholism and addiction, still held by many psychiatrists, may add to the high threshold which physicians must cross to become psychotherapy patients at an early stage of substance abuse. Effective early intervention in problems of alcohol and drug abuse by physicians will likely increase and thus call upon wider participation by psychiatrists in treatment. Psychotherapeutic issues, generally familiar to psychodynamically trained psychiatrists, have been reviewed with a focus on physicians in early phases of substance abuse. Particular attention is given, with case illustrations, to the therapeutic alliance, internal and external controls, and the need for specific concern with alcohol and drug dependency regardless of other associated factors in a given case. Psychotherapeutic aspects of treatment in more advanced stages of illness have also been briefly reviewed.

REFERENCES

1. Hall RCW, Stickney SK, Popkin MK: Physician drug abuser. *J Nerv Ment Disorder* 166:787–793, 1978.
2. Talbott, GD: The disabled doctors program of Georgia. *Alc: Clin Exp Res* 1:143–146, 1977.
3. Johnston GP: The impaired physician: A treatable problem. *J Ind State Med Assoc* 71:1058–1060, 1978.

4. Newson JA: Help for the alcoholic physician in California. *Alc: Clin Exp Res* 1:135–137, 1977.
5. Green RC, Carroll GJ, Buxton WD: Drug addiction among physicians: The Virginia experience. *JAMA* 236:1372–1375, 1976.
6. Gitlow SE: The disabled physician—his care in New York state. *Alc: Clin Exp Res* 1:131–134, 1977.
7. Dudley JC, Talbott GD: Disabled doctors program. Med Assoc of Georgia conference, Atlanta, Feb. 1977.
8. Bissell L, Jones RW: The alcoholic physician: A survey. *Am J Psychiat* 133:1142–1146, 1976.
9. Vaillant GE, Sobowale NC, McArthur C: Some psychologic vulnerabilities of physicians. *N Engl J Med* 287:372–375, 1972.
10. Modlin HC, Montes A: Narcotics addiction in physicians. *Am J Psychiat* 121:358–363, 1964.
11. Duffy JC, Litin EM: Psychiatric morbidity of physicians. *JAMA* 189:989–992, 1964.
12. Connelly JC: The alcoholic physician. *J Kans Med Soc* 79:601–604, 1978.
13. Anthony M: Al-Anon. *JAMA* 238:1062–1063, 1977.
14. Tokarz JP, Bremer W, Peters K, Pfifferling J-H, Viner J: *Beyond survival*. Resident Physician Section of the AMA, Chicago, 1979.
15. Lipsitt DR: The doctor as patient. *Psychiatric Opinion* 12: 20–25, 1975.
16. Johnson RP, Connelly JC: Addicted physicians: A closer look. *JAMA* 245:253–257, 1981.
17. Smith RJ, Steindler MS: The psychiatrist's role with the impaired physician. *Psychiatric Journal of the University of Ottawa* 7:3–7, 1982.
18. Arana GW: The impaired physician: a medical and social dilemma. *General Hospital Psychiatry* 4:147–154, 1982.
19. Herrington RE, Benzer DC, Jacobson GR, Hawkins MK: Treating substance-use disorders among physicians. *JAMA* 247:2253–2257, 1982.

IV

Special Problems in Treating Physicians

10

Responsibility, Confidentiality, and the Psychiatrically Ill Physician

BRIAN B. DOYLE

> These are the duties of a physician: First . . . to heal his mind and to give help
> to himself before giving it to anyone else.
>
> Athenian physician. A.D. 2[1]

Physicians are notoriously difficult patients, regardless of the type of their illness. It is particularly difficult for afflicted physicians, their family, friends, patients, and fellow physicians, to contend with psychiatric illness. Because of the emotional impact of psychiatric illness, the usual conflict between confidentiality and responsibility is heightened in those who would be helpful.

This chapter discusses the prevalence, etiologies, and treatment of psychiatric disorders in physicians. An investigation of the confidentiality–responsibility conflict leads to conclusions and recommendations for better prevention and treatment of these disorders.

THE PREVALENCE OF PSYCHIATRIC DISORDER IN PHYSICIANS

The true incidence of psychiatric disorder in physicians is elusive.[2-4] Estimates suggest that physicians suffer at least as much psychiatric illness as do other persons of comparable socioeconomic status.[2,5,6] For a variety of reasons they tend to have a higher incidence of affective disorder.[7] Physicians have a well-documented, higher suicide rate.[5,8-11] Studies of medical students, while not readily comparable with each other, show prevalence rates from 15% to 46% for significant psychiatric disorder.[2] Several anecdotal papers suggest that there is significant psychiatric disorder among resident physicians, with psychiatric residents the most frequently studied.[2] Reports on graduate physicians, while

BRIAN B. DOYLE • Department of Psychiatry and Behavioral Sciences, George Washington University School of Medicine and Health Sciences, Washington, D.C.

varied, support the impression of as much psychiatric disorder as among nonmedical peers.[1,5] Vaillant et al. reported on a longitudinal study of a cohort of 47 physicians and 79 controls through 30 years of adult life.[3] In their physician group 47% had bad marriages or divorce, 36% sought relief from drugs, 34% sought psychotherapy, and 17% had psychiatric hospitalization, all percentages significantly higher than in the controls. At least one other study, however, found that a cohort of California physicians had greater marital stability, with less divorce, separation, and annulment, than persons of similar age in the general population.[12]

Among physicians who become psychiatrically ill, clinicians generally are over-represented. Surgeons, researchers, and administrators are under-represented.[3,13] Controversy continues whether psychiatrists have a higher incidence of psychiatric illness generally, and of suicide specifically.[4,5] After reviewing the reports, Murray[13] stated finally that the evidence is not conclusive.

ETIOLOGY OF PSYCHIATRIC ILLNESS IN PHYSICIANS

Waring[2] cites the factors commonly held responsible for psychiatric illness in physicians: (1) the profession makes enormous demands; (2) drugs are readily available; (3) overwork and physician responsibility in life-and-death situations are extremely stressful; and (4) long medical training is itself stressful. While initially plausible, these arguments do not hold up; many other types of work are equally stressful, and many physicians thrive on the challenges. In one survey of 3946 primary-care physicians in the urban and suburban northeastern United States, of the 1156 M.D.s who responded, 169 (14.6%) had had psychotherapy.[14] There was no difference between physicians who had and who had not had psychotherapy in terms of the percentage of their time in clinical practice, in the number of weekly work hours (most worked more than 50 hours), or in the number of patients seen per day.

The consensus is that physicians with personality difficulties antedating medical school are vulnerable to the occupational hazards of a medical career.[2] Of physicians in the Vaillant et al. sample with good childhood adjustment, only 15% showed two or more psychiatric symptoms; the pecentage was 50% among those with poor childhood adjustment.[3] Psychiatric hospitalization in adulthood correlated well with poor childhood adjustment. Waring summarizes widely held views: "obsessionalism, lack of pleasure-seeking, and feelings of indispensability, while being useful as a student and fitting the 'good doctor' role, may predispose to affective disorders in middle life."[2] The term "masochism" repetitively occurs, and the decompensating physician is "harried, disorganized, and increasingly despairing."[2-4,6,15] Without the internal or social resources to meet the demands of his practice, he becomes increasingly depressed and withdrawn. While this is the general pattern in many physicians, others show severe problems. Examples are a surgeon who expressed his sadism by being overly pessimistic with patients, and a family physician who sexually abused little girls he examined while unchaperoned.[16] Sometimes the behavior is manifestly diagnosable. Examples are a surgeon who rewrote house officers' orders, believing they sought to humiliate him (paranoid schizophrenia); a psychiatrist who killed himself, leaving patients dangerously suicidal (psychotic depression); and a resident who falsified hematology and other laboratory data (antisocial personality).[16] Many physicians function remarkably well at work in spite of severe psychological difficulties.[2,17]

Physicians most commonly have psychiatric illness requiring hospitalization in their early to mid-40s, when they have been in practice for about 15 years.[2,3,7,14,18]

PHYSICIANS BECOMING PSYCHIATRIC PATIENTS

Several factors complicate ill physicians' seeking psychiatric help. Other medical professionals do not regard psychiatry highly as a specialty nor do physicians place much faith in the usefulness of psychiatric treatments.[19] In addition to having personality types which encourage avoidance and denial, many physicians self-diagnose and self-medicate. Most physicians who are not psychologically oriented will tend to experience emotional conflict as physical symptoms or attribute psychological distress to physical causes.[2]

The process by which physicians actually become psychiatric patients is often tortuous. Self-referral is unusual; family or peer pressure is commonly decisive.[1,18] Small et al. insist that colleagues are more instrumental in initiating and securing hospitalization than are the ill physicians or their family.[15] Far more typical is the assertion that colleagues are reluctant to take action, even when the physician is suffering severe mental illness.[4,16]

Where there are few doctors and the socio-economic levels are low, in some settings only colleagues may have sufficient status and prestige to confront the ill physician. Even then they may not do so. Enomoto cites an example where colleagues failed to respond to a drug-abusing physician. Only her repeated phone calls to a nonmedical friend prevented her dying from an overdose (personal communication). Often weeks or months of covert and increasingly anguished negotiations pass before the physician enters treatment. Those around the sick physician collude in his denial, minimizing the problems.[16]

Statistics about voluntary versus involuntary admissions of physicians give fresh evidence. In one study, 19.6% of physicians hospitalized for psychiatric illness were involuntary commitments, as opposed to 5.5% of controls.[20] Ross notes that many physicians fear loss of professional self-esteem more than loss of personal self-esteem. The reality of the psychiatric illness pales into insignificance compared to the threatened loss of his professional identity. The physician-patient's capacity to admit himself for treatment voluntarily is a good prognostic sign; few demonstrate this capacity. Admitting staff should explore, directly but tactfully, the physician-patient's feelings about hospitalization.[16]

PHYSICIANS IN TREATMENT

The physician's being in treatment, either as an inpatient or as an outpatient, precipitates a fresh round of struggles. Main's description[21] of "the special patient" fits psychiatrically ill physicians well: (1) a large proportion have medical connections; (2) they have shown some capacity for serving others at cost to themselves; (3) they are often admitted with pleas for special consideration; (4) they suffer intensely; and (5) the outcome is almost uniformly poor.

Physicians hospitalized in crisis will often reassert their denial and push for their accustomed dominance as soon as they begin to feel better.[7,16,18] A much higher proportion of physicians leave psychiatric hospitalization against medical advice than do other types of patients.[12,13,14] In one study, 1 in 8 physician-patients left against medical advice as opposed to 1 in 75 controls; in another, up to one-third of the physician-patients left against medical advice.[5,15] The characteristic struggles of the psychiatric inpatient are more intense with the ill physician.[1,14,16]

ISSUES FOR THERAPISTS WITH PSYCHIATRICALLY ILL PHYSICIANS

The most difficult problem for therapists is their identification with physician-patients.[2] Many psychiatrists become embarrassed and anxious when physician colleagues present themselves for treatment.[19] Anxiety resulting from a student's or physician's illness leads to collusion by the treating physician in the patient's denial. The results are under-diagnosis and insufficient treatment.[5,8] Treating psychiatrists protectively avoid diagnosing serious psychiatric disorders.[7,18] Some physicians who were former psychiatric patients, however, asserted that their psychiatrists over-estimated the severity of their disorders and under-estimated their resources.[15]

Psychiatrists mistakenly assume that other medical colleagues know about psychiatry. Often other physicians are not psychologically minded and are ignorant about psychiatric terminology, treatment goals, and methods.[2,7,14] Actively including the physician in his own management significantly improves outcome, according to principles of working with controlling patients advocated by Kahana and Bibring.[23] The physician with a coexisting or complicating illness especially challenges the psychiatrist. Unfamiliar with the classical medical problem, and upset by the manifestations of the patient's psychiatric illness, the treating psychiatrist is uncomfortable. Ross advocates a strong psychiatrist–internist alliance concerning management of general medical problems in the psychiatrically ill physician.[16]

Encounters with such patients are particularly difficult for the non-physician psychiatric staff.[16,18] They find it difficult to contend with the criticism, rationalizations, and projections of the sick doctor.[24] However, resourceful staff members can sidestep the ways psychiatrists and physician-patients lock horns over who's the "real" doctor.

The psychiatrist must also effectively mobilize human supports: family, colleagues, and friends. Families of physicians wish to see the spouse or parent as omnipotent again, and often prematurely.[16] They may collude in termination of treatment before it is appropriate. Cooperative colleagues often help ill physicians stay in treatment by maintaining the physician-patient's medical practice. Impaired physicians deeply appreciate this aid.[15] While physicians are often invested in helping colleagues return to function, this is not always the case.[17] At times the psychiatrist has a poor alliance with the family or with colleagues and must work alone to maintain the option that the physician-patient can resume practice. Such burdensome efforts are as necessary to successful treatment as are psychotherapeutic skills or appropriate medications.

THE RESULTS OF TREATMENT

No matter how expert the therapists, physician-patients tend to leave treatment earlier than recommended.[1,2,6,15,18] Some authors[1,2,13,14] assert that physicians do worse than nonphysician patients with similar diagnoses; others[6,15,16] claim they do better. Denial, rationalization, and escape back into work are cited as the major reasons why physicians do poorly. Ross[16] best expresses the optimistic view: "[The physician] brings to treatment many strengths and resources which, even though they may be hidden beneath his considerable resistance . . . can serve to reorient him to a better level of adjustment after psychiatric hospitalization."

According to Hoar et al.,[14] physicians who have had psychotherapy had more positive attitudes toward psychiatry. However, they had neither greater therapeutic skills nor more ease with psychiatric patients, nor did they make more referrals to psychiatrists.

Treatment has better results when it is in the context of official limitations which constitute "benign coercion."[13,15,17,24] Peer leverage, such as removing admission and operating privileges, effectively prompts the necessary hospital admission of the physician-patient.[7,18] In a 1973 report the AMA Council on Mental Health specified how a state medical society should organize peer leverage.[25] At that time, in the 37 societies reporting (of 54 surveyed) only 14 had active or pending programs, 23 had no program, and 3 denied any problems! Several states have since installed "sick doctor" laws, to provide the proper balance of coercive and noncoercive measures. As of February 1981 approximately 47 states had operating programs.[20]

In the past several years most states have been able to develop official programs. Although each state certainly should have one, more local, less official efforts may prove more useful.

Individual institutions have begun to develop mechanisms for caring for sick staff physicians. The Committee on Staff Health of the Institute of Pennsylvania Hospital, for example, offers confidential, expert and nondisciplinary help to physicians or their families. The committee recommends appropriate care while safeguarding the potential patient's staff position. Should this fail, their peer pressure can usefully be levied to prompt the disturbed physician to seek treatment.[7]

CONFIDENTIALITY VERSUS RESPONSIBILITY

The phrase "confidentiality versus responsibility" assumes that the two are in conflict. It is necessary to understand the origins and consequences of that assumption before better methods of prevention and intervention can be proposed for psychiatric illness in physicians.

Confidentiality is central to the physician's professional practice but the privilege by law is only partial. Nevertheless, we prize our personal conviction that what patients tell us is told in confidence. Physicians, including psychiatrists, have been willing to be imprisoned rather than betray a patient's confidence. Our concept includes appropriate sharing of information in supervision or with professional colleagues. Our ideals can make us excessively careful. At times we do not share information and concerns when desirable, thus remaining alone with our patients' grief and pain. Reticence about getting appropriate consultation and supervision can result in our being overwhelmed. Such self-imposed isolation could contribute to the high rate of physician suicide.

Psychiatric symptoms and illness are borne with shame, which medical professionals experience as well as laymen. Physicians who comfortably discuss intimate details of a patient's anatomy may lapse into troubled silence about that person's intimate life. The prohibitions on talking about patients operate more powerfully when we ourselves are the patient, and especially if our illness is psychiatric. According to Vaillant et al.,[3] the ill physician's defenses of reaction formation and altruism are expressed as "there's a lot wrong but I won't bother anyone with it." To do so would be to betray his patient's confidence, especially when the patient is himself! The sick physician covertly communicates this attitude to colleagues, who then feel constrained. They must not intrude on another physician's relationship with a patient, even if "the patient" is that physician.

Within this occult process lies its strength. Once these assumptions are explicit and open, they reveal themselves as illogical, emotional, and counter-productive. The sick physician's symptoms threaten the equilibrium of his colleagues.[2,14,16] Respecting the patient's privacy is laudable, but excessive concern for confidentiality hides an overestimation of our importance. At least in part grandiosity lies behind the reluctance of the ill physician to seek help and the reluctance of colleagues to intervene. To challenge a colleague's grandiosity is to confront our own.

Another element in the difficulties of physicians over referring a sick colleague is that we have conflicting responsibilities. We feel responsible not to label a friend as ill, nor to confront him unnecessarily. At the same time we feel responsible for a sick colleague's patients receiving adequate care. If his psychiatric illness is interfering with his providing proper medical care, then we feel pressed to intervene. That's difficult, knowing how precious a colleague's professional self-esteem is. "Responsibility versus responsibility" may well better explain the referring doctor's dilemma than "confidentiality versus responsibility."

At first glance the dictates of medical responsibility seem clear. The ill physician is responsible for seeking treatment, just as his colleagues are to help him. The responsibility of a physician often does not extend to ourselves or other physicians.[19] We tend to interpret "Physician, heal theyself!" as an order to self-diagnose and to treat; "Physician, care for thyself" would be more appropriate. Yet there is little reinforcement in medical education or professional life for the physician's caring for himself.

RECOMMENDATIONS FOR INTERVENTION

Successful treatment programs for psychiatrically ill physicians require a balance of voluntary and benign coercive methods.[20,24] However effective, they are tertiary prevention, and we need to consider earlier interventions.

Vaillant et al. propose that physicians who develop psychiatric illness usually have a history of difficulties preceding medical school.[3] Psychiatric screening of applicants' records or of the applicants themselves is possible, and already has been proposed in Great Britain.[13] The predictive value of such screening is unproven. Eliciting a history of successful coping with life difficulties in medical school applicants is a more positive approach, but the demands on the time and energy of overworked admissions committees would be unrealistic. Further, screening proposals ignore the attitude of free will which permeates the medical profession.[2]

The process of gaining entry into medical school fosters competition and self-sufficiency in students, qualities which most medical schools tolerate or actively encourage. But if "physicians need permission to cherish themselves and to admit that they have needs,"[3] medical school is a good place to begin to learn how. Faculty and administrators who agree can implement programs in the official curriculum which embody this principle. A comprehensive student health service, providing ready access to total health care, is a prerequisite. All schools do not have such a service. Such a lack dramatizes the failure of medical schools to acknowledge and implement this principle.[5] Another mechanism is faculty-run student groups which include mutual support among their objectives. Doyle and others have run elective "Identity of the Physician" groups for medical students.[30] At the same medical school, Webster and Robinowitz have reported on a 4-year experience with such an identity group.[31] The students sustained their work, not just through the usual trials of medical school, but also through the psychiatric illness of one of the members. Experience is similar at other medical schools: elective enrollment tends to increase, and students profit by group leaders who are nonpsychiatrists and psychiatrists.

The groups reported on by Webster and Robinowitz, and Doyle, are voluntary electives; one can object that they reach the students who need them least. Williams and his co-workers, in contrast, make small-group participation mandatory for all medical students throughout their first year. Psychiatrists and other physicians lead the groups, which students generally like. Some leaders have been surprised and moved at how powerfully their student groups support them (personal communication). Making such experiences mandatory may diminish their value, since the requirement increases student resistance. The skillful group leader will expect and explore student resistance to a group designed for mutual help and sustenance. Another objection is that such group experiences unnecessarily "psychiatrize" students. Having non-psychiatric as well as psychiatric leaders may meet this objection. More effective is the direct approach: being generally healthy, students can learn about and develop mature interdependence. Having such groups as an official part of the curriculum, implemented by the administration and not sponsored by departments of psychiatry alone, reinforces that these concerns are schoolwide, not just psychiatric. Although the groups have a good theoretical rationale, Waring points out that their value is unproven.[2] "Happiness" data do not prove impact on the participants' current or future life.

Many psychiatric training programs have included mandatory small-group experiences for residents, particularly in the first year. While these have focused primarily on understanding group dynamics or social systems, mutual support in a stressful time has been a secondary function. Max Day, at the Massachusetts Mental Health Center, and Roger Shapiro, at George Washington University Medical Center, led such groups for many years. Only a few programs require such an experience and openly encourage its supportive functions. The difficulties psychiatrists have fostering healthy interdependence is all the more striking because educators regard the first year of residency as particularly stressful.

Some family practice programs such as the one at the Medical College of South Carolina have made small-group experiences integral parts of the residency. Social and professional isolation will be a difficult problem for family practitioners, especially in areas which are rural or underserved or both. An explicit objective is to develop a support group which will persist when the residents are in practice. While it is early yet to test the operational effectiveness of such a plan, its theoretical advantages are considerable.

American Psychiatric Association leaders have recently sponsored measures which are useful, practical, and encouraging. Surveys for preferences in continuing education show that APA members strongly favor small-group settings where active learning and peer supervision can take place (personal communication). When suitably planned and organized, small groups are now eligible for Category I credit toward continuing education requirements. In successful groups the mutual support and supervision which evolves naturally can be as valuable as the formal learning. This is an imaginative first step in what is a vital process: not just finding ways to care for ourselves and each other, but rewarding ourselves and each other for so doing.

SUMMARY

In summary, psychiatrically ill physicians are often reluctant and uncooperative patients. Efforts to help them are conflict-ridden and difficult. Powerful assumptions about confidentiality and responsibility impede effective intervention. Inappropriately regarding himself as his own patient, the sick doctor guards his confidentiality, acting to preserve his sense of being invulnerable. Their own equilibrium threatened, colleagues respond with denial and avoidance. Successful intervention requires programs which combine voluntary action and benign coercion. That 47 states now have operational programs testifies to a breakthrough in the conflicts between confidentiality and responsibility. "Physician, care for thyself" may be more useful dictum than "Physician, heal thyself." This is contrary to strong traditional assumptions.

To be most successful, programs from medical school to continuing education must contain the following elements:

1. They are official programs required for all trainees.
2. In nonpsychiatric settings, nonpsychiatrists as well as psychiatrists have administrative and operational responsibility.
3. "Learning to sustain ourselves and each other" is an acknowledged goal, not simply inferred or assumed.
4. The style and substance meet the expressed preferences of the physicians involved.
5. Physicians are positively reinforced (e.g., by getting Category I Continuing Medical Education credits) for their participation.

REFERENCES

1. Duffy JC, Litin, EM: Psychiatric morbidity of physicians. *JAMA* 189:989–992, 1964.
2. Waring EM: Psychiatric illness in physicians: A review. *Psychiat* 15:519–520, 1974.

3. Vaillant GC, Sobowale NC, McArthur C: Some psychologic vulnerabilities of physicians. *N Engl J Med* 287:372–375, 1972.
4. Scheiber S: Emotional problems of physicians. *Ariz Med* 34:323–325, 1977.
5. a'Brook MF, Hailstone JD, McLauchlan IEJ: Psychiatric illness in the medical profession. *Br J Psychiat* 113:1013–1023, 1967.
6. Pearson MM, Strecker EA: Physicians as psychiatric patients: Private practice experience. *Am J Psychiat* 116:915–919, 1960.
7. Jones RE: A study of 100 physician psychiatric inpatients. *Am J Psychiat* 134:1119–1123, 1977.
8. Pond DA: Doctor's mental health (ed), Mental disturbance in doctors. *NZ Med J* 69:131–135, 1969.
9. Sainsbury P: Suicide and depression, in Coppen AJ, Walk A (eds): *Recent Developments in Affective Disorders*. London, Headley Brothers, 1968, pp 1–33.
10. Simon W, Lumry GK: Suicide among physician-patients. *J. Nerv Ment Disorder* 147:105–112, 1968.
11. Jones RE: Physician's personality a factor in psychiatric hospitalization. *Roche Rep: Frontiers in Psychiatry* April 15, 1977.
12. Rose KD, Rosow I: Physicians who kill themselves. *Arch Gen Psychiat* 29:800–805, 1973.
13. Murray M: Psychiatric illness in doctors. *Lancet* 1:1211–1213, 1974.
14. Haar E, Green MR, Hyams L: Characteristics of physicians who have had psychotherapy. *Arch Gen Psychiat* 27:705–709, 1972.
15. Small IF, Small JG, Assue CM, et al: Fate of the mentally ill physician. *Am J Psychiat* 125:1333–1342, 1969.
16. Ross JL: The physician as a psychiatric patient. *Psychiat Digest* 37:46, 1971.
17. Shapiro ET, Pinsker H, Shale JH: The mentally ill physician as practitioner. *JAMA* 232:725–727, 1975.
18. Gold N: The doctor, his illness, and the patient. *Aust NZ J Psychiat* 6:209–213, 1972.
19. Menninger RW: Mental health and the physician: Who worries about his? *Maryland State Med J* 19:58–62, 1970.
20. Robertson J. Report of the American Medical Association Council of Mental Health, March 1981.
21. Main T: The ailment. *Brit J Med Psychiat* 30:129–145, 1957.
22. Kahana R, Bibring G: Personality types in medical management, in Zinberg N (ed): *Psychiatry and Medical Practice in a General Hospital*, New York, International Universities Press, 1964, pp 108–123.
23. Pollack IW, Battle WC: Studies of the special patient. *Arch Gen Psychiat* 9:344–350, 1963.
24. Impaired physicians now may find help through MSMS program, editorial: *Mich Med* 37:413–420, 1975.
25. AMA Council on Mental Health: The sick physician: Impairment by psychiatric disorders. *JAMA* 223:684–687, 1973.
26. Webster TG, Robinowitz CB: Medical student identity group: A four year experience. Paper presented at the Annual Meeting of the American Psychiatric Association, Toronto, Canada, May 4, 1977.

11

The Physician as a Patient

CAROLYN B. ROBINOWITZ

One of the most pervasive medical myths involves doctors as patients. Traditionally there have been aphorisms and injunctions from biblical times until the present: "Physician heal thyself!" "The doctor who treats himself has a fool for a patient!" The standard hospital stock statement is that doctors and nurses make the worst patients, possibly because there are no surprises left for them in hospitals.

Why is there the feeling that, like the shoemaker's barefoot children, the doctor and his or her family often receive the worst medical care? What is there about physicians, in terms of their background, expectations, knowledge, attitudes, and skills that creates and perpetuates this "worst patient" syndrome? Are doctors poorer risks if they are ill? Are they prone to be more concerned about prevention, changes in life style, or early intervention? Are they usually in better health than other hardworking professionals? Do they enter the hospital in poorer condition due to delay and/or lack of personal concern? Do they really have bad care in hospitals, and is there a basic underlying truth about that "worst patient" folklore?[1]

A study in the *New England Journal of Medicine* demonstrated that graduate students received more adequate health care than did house staff.[2,3] Most nonmedical students have some access to comprehensive student health plans and usually consider the purchase of health insurance. There is a much more cavalier attitude by and toward physician-students or house staff. Medical student health plans are less organized (especially for prevention). It is assumed that because of professional courtesy, doctors do not need comprehensive medical insurance plans. Perhaps part of the physicians' reluctance to obtain checkups or request medical care early in the course of an illness may be due to their lack of experience with regular, systematic health care.

CAROLYN B. ROBINOWITZ • Deputy Medical Director, American Psychiatric Association, Washington, D.C.

Other studies of physician and medical student experiences support the psychological view. Doctors are afraid of death and disease, and work very hard to combat it. This usually appropriate effort can lead to extraordinary approaches to the care and cure of patients. In medical school, death is seen as an enemy to be feared and challenged. Physicians, through engaging in the battle, and frequently winning, support their own fantasies of immortality. Like the tightrope walker who has conquered heights, physicians may use their own knowledge and skills to defend themselves against their own anxiety about strength, body integrity, and dangers of illness and death.[4,5]

A sizable number of medical students or their families have experienced serious or potentially life-threatening illness during childhood. For many of them, therefore, identification with an idealized god-like and caring physician who provides succor, healing, and empathy is related to their personal quest for an idealized omnipotent caring parent. Becoming a physician can evoke a way of identifying with and incorporating the care-giver, thus supporting dependency needs while giving strength and power. For others, the sense of identification with the aggressor is marked. In either situation, a feeling of weakness on the part of the embryo physician is almost intolerable. A common childhood experience—especially for boys—was the admonition to "grin and bear it," avoiding giving in to pain or injury and with much admiration of the person who was strong.[6,7] Certainly the folklore of medical school abounds with anecdotes of physicians who kept going no matter what, enduring sleep deprivation, long hours of work, and performing even when personally ill. The stories of doctors who left their sickbeds immediately following their own surgery to take care of another, more urgently ill patient are not just apocryphal. Rather, they are ingrained into the medical student culture and serve as models to be emulated.

It may be that physicians who recommend preventive health care, such as regular diet, no smoking, moderation in alcohol consumption, cardiovascular-related exercise, adequate rest, spaced vacations, and freedom from stress, do not personally indulge in this caretaking behavior. They may view such concerns magically or as being based on old wives' tales without personal import, in spite of supporting scientific data. For the physician who is committed to the magic or protection of the doctor's role, no special precautions are needed.[8]

Physical illness brings with it a real pain and limitation of activities, as well as a tremendous narcissistic threat to the fantasy of omnipotence and immortality.[8] A not unusual comment made by physician-patients in intensive care or coronary care units is "How could *I* get *sick*?" It is uttered with a total sense of disbelief which verges on denial. The impact of illness becomes devastating. The magic has slipped away, and the doctor may be left overwhelmed by feelings of helplessness and inadequacy, which are all the more troubling because of the perceived loss of the magical protection. Attempts at reconstitution involve denial, reaction formation, and other defenses, and the physician-patient may subsequently get up too soon or return to unhealthy habit patterns. Such actions predispose to illness in an attempt to "prove" the return of power. It is difficult for the physician-patient to admit to fear, feelings of weakness, loss, or inadequacy, missing an opportunity to ventilate feelings, with cathartic relief.[9]

Some physician-patients become so overwhelmed by their illness that they regress to a more primitive manner of coping. They may become overly dependent, clinging, depressed, suspicious, and even paranoid. They need immediate intervention to help them deal with the crisis that led to their loss of power, control, as well as body functioning involved in their illness.

The physician-patient may resist the dependency that illness brings with it and refuse to let the caring physician provide care. The treating physician may vacillate between permissiveness and authoritarian control. Roles become blurred, and it is often difficult to distinguish who is doing the "doctoring." This role blurring is an issue, because the patient who is ill and in need, or who becomes temporarily dependent and passive, and the doctor in charge, who may become intrusive and controlling in caring for the patient, function in a relationship that only occurs during illness. The doctor may ask and hear about very personal material, see parts of the body rarely if ever viewed publicly, and in the interest of helping the patient temporarily control all the patient's activities, causing regression as well as pain and distress.[10]

It is implicit in this relationship that doctors possess certain skills and knowledge, and the patient must maintain some degree of trust and willingness. However, when the patient is a physician, additional problems may occur. The patient is often conflicted by the traditional need to know, to be in charge, and to control the course of medical treatment, as opposed to the need to relinquish this to the caretaking physician. The patient swings between being colleague, friend, and collaborator to demanding, difficult patient.

Although physicians may not be such different patients medically, they are treated differently by those responsible for their care. They, themselves, may insist upon and require different care. Special meals, rooms, and visiting privileges are common for doctors who are ill. The treating physician, too, may be aware of inner feelings of uneasiness and resentment, and find it difficult to treat the patient in the usual manner.

Defensive, and sensing the patient's close scrutiny of case management, the doctor tends to be cautious and much more conservative. The therapeutic relationship and the manner and method with which the two relate will be colored by mutual anxiety and insecurities in the roles of physician and patient.[11,12]

The physician-patients' medical knowledge may indeed contribute to their anxiety and lack of cooperation. Doctors generally have very strong feelings of knowledge and control, and as a group physicians are resistant to changes in habits, practice pattern, etc.*

In addition, there is always some degree of suspicion or lack of trust about the practice habits of colleagues. Some clearly cynical people have suggested that the suspicion is related to doctors' intimate knowledge of colleagues' lack of perfection and the things that can go wrong—something often kept hidden from the general public.[13] That would seem to be only a portion of the cause of suspicion. The less rational aspect may relate to physicians' own loss of fantasied omniscience or omnipotence in becoming a patient, as well as lack of success in curing their own ills.[14,15]

This anxiety may influence choice of personal physicians. There is a fallacy in the concept that the doctor with many physician-patients is the most competent. Bynder noted that over 75% of physicians, when choosing a personal physician, tend to choose someone they knew previously, who is not necessarily the most competent or respected. About half of the choices studied were based on a friendship or a social relationship rather than professional competence. Thus the doctor-patient attempts to avoid anxiety or the unknown, but in so doing may receive less than optimal care.[16,17]

The personal-social quality of the doctor–patient relationship creates another problem. Friends who are anxious not to cause discomfort or stress tend to avoid often needed but unpleasant or painful procedures. The deferred pelvic and rectal examinations may spare embarrassment, but may also allow the cancer to remain dormant. Bone marrow examinations may be delayed. Both parties may "know" what is being avoided, but there is a subtle, covert agreement to "cover up" and "be nice," while both are anxious, and even guilty, about this special treatment.

---

* E.g., education to new drug therapies has only minimal impact on performance patterns unless the education takes place in the clinical setting and is reinforced. Although physicians may gain a great deal of knowledge about a drug, they tend not to prescribe it, tending to continue to use drugs they know well.

Professional courtesy, while traditionally demanded, adds to the difficulty. It underscores the familial and social aspects of the doctor–patient relationship while creating obstacles to good care. No longer is a service purchased; instead, something is being given. The effect is that the patient becomes hesitant or guilty about disturbing a colleague, and delays calls and appointments. Consultation may come through a telephone call, not a visit. Treatment may be prescribed without a thorough examination. The physician-patient is limited in expressing disagreement or dissatisfaction with the care provided, by virtue of being the recipient of this "free" time and attention. One response is to "take over" and self-prescribe rather than to express anger or disappointment.[18]

The factors involved in physician-patienthood are complex.[19-22] Many physicians honestly believe they want their doctor to take total responsibility for their care. However, there are too many obstacles to hurdle in order to make that wish a reality. Treating physicians are anxious about their own skills and knowledge, and may therefore, treat physician-patients as colleagues who can provide consultation and collaboration in this "interesting case." This inappropriate inclusion of the physician-patient in case discussion and management is further complicated by the diminution of judgment that occurs with the anxiety, the investment of physician-patients in their own care, and issues of countertransference. At this point decision-making is no longer an entirely rational process. The problem increases when the physician-patient's specialty is not in the area of the illness, or lack of knowledge compounds the communication problem, since the physician-patient may not be as able to understand the differential diagnosis or treatment plan rationally and needs to be treated more like a nonmedical patient.

A more subtle problem develops if the treating physician has difficulty maintaining the image of knowledgeable, god-like, omnipotent healer. No longer can the patient's expectations help rather than hinder the treatment process.[23] The patient may well remember that the treating physician was in the lower half of medical school class, gave a poor presentation at grand rounds, or had personal problems. The treating physician thus begins care from a defensive stance, and the usual patient expectation that the care will "work," and that cure will follow, is tempered by harsh reality and often doomed to failure.

While for many physicians this experience can bring about a greater understanding of their own role in the experience of patienthood, it can be a costly lesson, deleterious to the health of all concerned. These issues might better be learned in a more protected setting—one in which life and health were not at stake.

Many medical schools have developed simulated experiences for student physicians, and some have used an intensive plan to promote preventive health care for their students as a way of bringing these issues into focus. One school, for example,[24] developed a plan by which medical students were exposed to an extremely comprehensive and thoughtful prevention program, consisting of health evaluation, immunization, and prescription of activities and behavior consistent with maintaining good health or improving current problems. Rather than experiencing this in isolation, students participated in it as part of a formal course on the role of the patient and physician. Consequently students read and discussed literature on the styles and functions of physicians, and identified what they wanted from their physicians and from medical care in general. The entire practical experience as patients was then discussed and processed by both sets of participants—medical students and participating physician faculty. This was followed by comments from a variety of medical behavioral scientists. This unique combination of practical "real life" experience with cognitive follow-up provided needed increased sensitivity and insight into issues of health care. It also created an ongoing and continuous process and model for monitoring student health care throughout medical school. These students planned to be more active participants in their own health care. It was postulated that they would more actively involve their own patients in maintaining individual health care at a later time.

Awareness of the psychological determinants that each student brings to medical school allows for earlier intervention and an opportunity for each student to face the painful disappointment that comes with recognition of limits and loss of fantasied omnipotence. In addition the student can identify the various facets of the role of the physician in a more realistic way.[25]

Identity groups have supported such understanding and development, and student physicians who participate in them tend to find medical school a less dehumanizing experience.[26-28] Webster and Robinowitz reported on a long-term student group attended by medical students in their last 3 years of training.[29] Although the group had an initial explicit emphasis on professional identity and physicianhood, the group provided a core around which both clinical training and personal psychotherapeutic content and process were woven. The participants at a 10-month follow-up felt they had a deeper understanding of themselves as persons and physicians, increasing competence in their clinical competencies and career direction, plus solutions to emotional problems and prevention, biases, and narrow attitudes often reinforced by the medical school experience. We would assume that these students would be better able to integrate the psychological and physical aspects of medical care with their own role and identity as care providers.

Such integrating experiences provide opportunity for personal and professional growth and development, and allow the physician to be a better patient and a better care-giver.

REFERENCES

1. Pinner M, Miller BF: *When Doctors Are Patients*. New York, Norton. 1952.
2. Heller RJ, Robertson LS, Alpert JJ: Health care of house officers: A comparative study. *N Engl J Med* 277:907–910, 1967.
3. House staffs without coverage. *N Engl J Med* 277:934–935, 1967.
4. Oker D: The doctor's job: An update. *Psychosomat Med* 40:449–461, 1978.
5. Pitts FN Jr, Winokur G, Steward MA: Psychiatric syndromes, anxiety, symptoms, and responses to stress in medical students. *Am J Psychiat* 118:333–340, 1961.
6. Merton RK: Some preliminaries to a sociology of medical education, in Merton R, Reader G, Kendall P (eds): *The Student Physician*, Cambridge, Mass., Harvard University Press, 1957, pp 3–80.
7. Becker HS, Geer B, Hughes EC, et al: *Boys in White—Student Culture in Medical School*. Chicago, University of Chicago Press, 1961, pp 419–435.
8. Grotjahn M: On being a sick physician, in Wahl C (ed): *New Dimensions in Psychosomatic Medicine*, Boston, Little Brown, 1964.
9. Pinner M: My cardiac disease, in Pinner M, Miller BF: *When Doctors Are Patients*, New York, Norton, 1952.
10. Henderson LJ: Physician and patient as a social system. *N Engl J Med* 212:819–823, 1935.
11. Vincent MO, Robinson EA, Latt L: Physicians as patients: Private psychiatric hospital experience. *Can Med Assoc J* 100:403–412, 1969.
12. Pearson MM, Streaker EA: Physicians as psychiatric patients: Private practice experience. *Am J Psychiat* 116:915–919, 1960.
13. Lublin JS: Do doctors need a check-up? *Wall Street Journal*, Feb. 25, 1974.
14. Dowling HF: Physician, heal thyself. *G P* 11:69–73, 1955.
15. Crosbie S: The doctor as a patient. *Rocky Mt Med J* 69:49–52, 1962.
16. Bynder H: How does an ailing M.D. pick a doctor? *Med World*, Nov. 24, 1967.
17. Bynder H: Physicians choose psychiatrists: Medical social structure and patterns of choice. *J Health Hum Behav* 6:83–91, 1965.
18. Crawshaw RS: Who is my brother's keeper? *Federation Bull* 58:364–372, 1871.
19. Zabaranko RN, Zabarenko C, Pittenger RA: The psychodynamics of physicianhood. *Psychiatry* 33:102–118, 1970.
20. Parsons T: Illness and the role of the physician: A sociological perspective. *Am J Orthopsychiat* 21:452–460, 1951.
21. Lewin BD: Counter-transference in the technique of medical practice. *Psychosomat Med* 8:195–199, 1966.
22. Nunberg H: Psychological interrelations between physician and patient. *Psychoanalyt Rev* 25:197–308, 1938.
23. Frank JD: *Persuasion and Healing*, 2nd ed. Baltimore, Johns Hopkins Press, 1973.

24. Robinowitz CB: Health ecology: Teaching medical students psychosocial factors in health care for themselves and their patients. Unpublished paper, 1972.

25. Airing CD: Sympathy and empathy. *JAMA* 167:448–452, 1968.

26. Eron L: Effects of medical education on attitudes. *J Med Educ* 10:559–566, 1955.

27. Eron L: The effect of medical education on attitudes: A follow-up study. *J Med Educ* 33:25–33, 1958.

28. Rezler AG: Attitude changes during medical school: A review of the literature. *J Med Educ* 49:1023–1030, 1974.

29. Webster TG, Robinowitz CB: Becoming a physician: Long term student group. *J Gen Hosp Psychiat* 3:53–61, 1979.

V

The Impaired Physician
A Collective Responsibility

12

The Impaired Physician and Organized Medicine

CAROLYN B. ROBINOWITZ

It has been estimated that 5%–12% of the physicians in the United States are impaired sufficiently that their condition affects their work and practice. The most common diagnoses are alcohol and drug abuse, emotional disorders, illness related to aging and loss, or physical conditions.[1] While traditionally recognition and care of these physicians has been seen as the responsibility of the profession, the lack of success of voluntary treatment, and the inability of many medical groups to initiate effective limiting and/or disciplinary action has led to the increasing concern and involvement of the public, governmental groups (e.g., licensing bodies), as well as organized groups of physicians. A study performed by the American Medical Association stressed that ignorance, apathy, and a lack of feelings of responsibility by physicians generally existed in regard to the impaired and incompetent physician, with intervention coming late in the course of events, or even after the fact (as in physician suicide).[2] There are numerous and complex reasons for such delay or inaction.[3,4]

Organized medicine has made great strides in handling the problems of the impaired physician and is beginning to consider primary and secondary prevention. There are techniques available for early intervention and prevention of deterioration and/or suicide. Nonetheless psychosocial barriers remain which interfere with intervention and remediation, and individual attempts often fail.[5]

Since the manifestations of impairment are often subtle, problems are seldom recognized at an early stage. Physicians can often conceal the impact of their disability until it is quite severe, and the isolation and relative lack of peer review in practice delays the process of recognition.

CAROLYN B. ROBINOWITZ ● Deputy Medical Director, American Psychiatric Association, Washington, D.C.

In addition there is reluctance of family and friends to intervene. Physicians are afraid to point a finger at colleagues with whom they deal on a social and professional basis ("let he who is without sin . . .") and tend to deny signs and symptoms until they are more overtly disabling.[6]

There are several levels at which organized medicine has responded to needs of impaired physicians. These range from committees formed in local hospitals ("staff health and well-being committees") to the more formal activities of national organizations, state medical societies, or state licensing boards. The roles and functions vary. Support functions, including advocacy, confrontation, education, and assistance, are most effective with early problem recognition. Other groups are disciplinary or authoritarian, and remove a troubled physician from the practice of medicine until the impairment is under control.

The American Medical Association, recognizing the increasing problem of losing productive physicians due to varying types of impairment and the impact of their disability on the quality of patient care, has taken an active leadership role in activities related to this condition. The AMA's first formal program, "The Disabled Doctor: A Challenge to the Profession," was held in April, 1975 in San Francisco. A follow-up program in 1977, "The Impaired Physician: Answering the Challenge," was successful. The third program in 1978 dealt with special kinds of problems such as the aged physician, problems of female physicians, medical marriages, and aspects of caring for impaired residents and medical students. The AMA has focused on legal aspects of impairment, structure and function of state medical society and licensing board programs, hospital programs, confrontation techniques, treatment techniques, advocacy for the disabled doctor, and the role of auxiliary groups. These meetings have served as an impetus to create more effective state and local intervention programs.[7]

The fourth program in 1980, "Threshold '80: Building Well-Being," was co-sponored by the Medical Chirurgical Society of Maryland and focused on prevention and well-being. Medical school deans, students, house staff representatives, and residents joined with a series of experts to discuss topics such as the aging physician, curriculum development, hospital and medical society programs, legal aspects of impairment, psychiatric case finding, and student and resident well-being. Workshop groups emphasized stress management in medical school and residency, how to help fellow students or residents in trouble, the problems of special population groups, e.g., women, older students, homosexual students or residents, and racial minorities. In a workshop dealing with "things they didn't teach me in medical school," participants discussed events and situations of professional and family life that contribute to impairment, including leisure time, income, and specialty choice.

A key part of the conference dealt with confrontation techniques for case finding, persuading colleagues to seek help, as well as retraining and liaison between state medical societies and specialty societies.

A Staff Advisory Committee on Prevention of Impairment in Physicians in Training was recently organized by the AMA Department of Mental Health. Staff members from the Departments of Medical Student Affairs, Housestaff Affairs, Hospitals, Undergraduate and Graduate Medical Education participated in planning activities in the areas of prevention, treatment, and rehabilitation of medical students and residents impaired by substance abuse and mental illness.

The AMA Department of Mental Health has also been instrumental in developing a model act to be used by any state considering legislation relative to physician licensure. This act incorporated responsiblity of the physician for monitoring his/her own ethics. The AMA has also published the *Impaired Physician Newsletter,*[8] and has compiled a bibliography on the impaired physician (see Appendix B).

In 1981 a panel on the impaired physician—a component of the Council of Scientific Affairs—was formed to study issues of physician suicide and illness. The American Medical Student Association has studied impairment, and in March, 1981 sponsored a national conference, "Medical Student Well-Being: Towards Prevention of Impairment," with a focus on developmental aspects of being a medical student, peer responsbility, "life after medical school," and establishing support systems.

Curriculum development, issues of stress as in the medical marriage, special vulnerabilities of women, minorities, and white men, aspects of substance abuse, and confidentiality and due process were discussed in workshops. AMSA promotes use of support groups, peer counseling, and improved student health services to deal with these problems.

The American Psychiatric Association noted the interest in physician illness, and in 1979 the president appointed a Task Force on the Impaired Physician. This task force is housed in the Council on Medical Education and Career Development, as it is felt that education is vital not only for early identification and treatment but to provide information, knowledge, awareness, and options for improving lifestyles and practice activities to prevent stress, anxiety, and impairment.

The task force has collected information from district branches as to their activities for impaired colleagues and prepared a package of informational materials on program development. Members of the task force are charged to work with the AMA in a pilot project on the study of physician suicide through the use of postmortem interviews of survivors and colleagues. While goals remain heavily focused on identification and early and appropriate intervention, efforts will also be geared to determining particular patterns in development, lifestyle, and practice that are more apt to lead to difficulty as well as ways to provide needed educational experiences.

Forty-five state medical associations have authorized the formation of definitive programs to aid impaired physicians. They vary from those which are completely voluntary to more mandatory ones. In voluntary programs, a physician who is brought to the attention of the state medical association can receive help if he is willing. If he refuses help, little or nothing is done. The mandatory programs require reports to be sent to the state medical association and/or to the licensing board.

The author queried 51 state medical societies and state licensing boards to obtain information on their procedures and programs for the impaired physician. Their responses (50 state medical societies and 45 licensing boards) form the basis for the information described hereafter. The specific information on each state is available upon request from the author (see also Appendix A).

IMPAIRED PHYSICIAN COMMITTEES

Some states have an around-the-clock hotline for reporting concerns, with the anonymity of the caller guaranteed (although callers will be asked for identification). This report will then be referred to the committee without identifying the reporting person.

The initial request for assistance may come from the hospital staff, local medical societies, family, or friends. The first responsibility of the committee is to verify, in a discrete manner, whether the physician is troubled. The physician is then approached by one or more members of the committee who make up a contact team and who gently confront the physician with how others perceive his problem, suggest he seek help, and offer assistance. They attempt to motivate the physician toward treatment as well as protect him from the embarrassment and hardship incident to the illness, assist the physician in reentry to practice following the completion of treatment, and finally, act as friends or advocates for the physician in relationships, governmental agencies, and the board of medical practice.

Membership on the committees varies. In some states members' names are kept confidential to avoid coercion and to maintain committee privacy. Most specialties are represented, and age, gender, geographic location, and ethnic background are considered. There are representations of physicians with expertise in substance abuse, emotional disorders, and geriatrics. Many committees also include some rehabilitated formerly impaired M.D.'s.

In general, the membership does not include officers or any members with disciplinary or licensing powers, since their presence may deter requests for help from those who fear being involved in disciplinary action. A committee cannot serve two masters; that is, it cannot have a treating and disciplinary function. Within legal limits, the committee should provide clear and credible assurances of inviolable confidentiality if it is to help.

The committees carry out the objectives in a discrete and confidential manner, with an effort to dispel the "conspiracy of silence" that prevents friends, colleagues, spouses and family, hospital personnel, and others from reporting impaired physicians. Their approach is described as compassionate, concerned, caring, nonjudgmental advocacy.

After investigating the situation, the contact team plans an approach to the troubled doctor that is appropriate to the circumstances. An interview can provide the best approach to unearth evidence of symptoms and suggest recommendations. Thus if the physician is emotionally disturbed or suicidal, the psychiatrist member may be of great help in planning an unabrasive productive intervention.

The responsibility of the contact team is to induce the physician to enter treatment. The presence of two or three members provides support in a potentially tense situation and emphasizes the serious concern about the physician's peformance and welfare. There can be a second team and visit if the first is unsuccessful. If the physician agrees to enter treatment, the contact team requests that he sign an informal contract agreeing to enter and complete treatment, and to be monitored by the committee following the completion of treatment for a period of time deemed necessary by the committee. If the physician is not willing to enter treatment, then the team will inform him that he may be reported to the board of trustees of the medical society. They have the responsibility of deciding whether the matter should be brought to the attention of the board of medical practice. In this instance, the Committee for the Impaired Physician will terminate its official relationship with the physician, but can be available in an advocacy role, if the (refusing) physician should seek its help in the future.

Changes in laws requiring physicians to report impaired physicians to the medical board have aided in detection while raising problems about confidentiality. The obligation to report can interfere with anonymity and confidentiality.

Committees combine concerns for treatment, which must be confidential for the physician-patient to utilize it, with monitoring, which may be legally as well as ethically required. Clearly, a sick physician who continues to act out with alcohol, drug abuse, or in other ways will not feel free to admit these behaviors to a person who may have to report him. Also, it is difficult to trust a therapist to whom one has been assigned, yet a free choice of reporting physician may well lead the sick physician to choose a friend who may be more lenient.[9] A solution to this problem is to assign the job of monitor to a physician who would agree to fill the role but who would not perform treatment. Thus the treating physician would not breach the confidence of the physician-patient, while the monitor has responsbility to determine whether or not the sick physician's behavior prevents his continuing in the practice of medicine without endangering the welfare of his patients. The monitor, who should be very knowledgeable about treatment, would be assigned, while the sick physician would have free choice of the person to conduct treatment. The medical treatment would be at the suggestion of the committee or medical board, and monitoring would permit a prompt resolution of disciplinary actions without interfering with treatment.

Medical boards tend to be more involved in disciplinary actions, especially if there is no referral procedure or if the physician refuses voluntary treatment. Many licensing boards have statutory authority to suspend or limit medical licenses temporarily (or for a limited amount of time) without notice or hearing if the board believes that a cause exists for such suspension or limitation and that the licensee's continuation of practice would constitute a danger to the public health and safety. Simultaneously the board must institute proceedings for a hearing by the licensee. The board can require a physical and/or mental examination as well. State boards can prosecute cases in a manner similar to civil litigation.

STATE PLANS

Pennsylvania has developed an approach through cooperation of the medical society and licensing board. The impaired physician committee directs educational efforts to appropriate groups, established a registry of the best appropriate resources and therapies in the areas of substance abuse, mental health, and geriatrics, and updates it as necessary. Thus the committee supplies factual information concerning these conditions, makes knowledgeable referrals for effective treatment, confirms complaints, and refers them to an intervention team. It evaluates the degree of impairment in relation to the quality and efficiency of services rendered by physicians referred to the committee, recommends overall policy, develops guidelines regarding the implementation and maintenance of the program, reviews follow-up information, and makes recommendations if their attempts meet with failure.

The Pennsylvania intervention team members are selected for their expertise; they may themselves be rehabilitated impaired physicians. The team is not involved in the ongoing treatment process, but rather meets with the impaired physician with documentation that the impairment exists, expresses the concerns of colleagues, and encourages the impaired physician voluntarily to seek help or active treatment. The intervenors maintain contact to support and encourage cooperation, make every effort to assist the impaired physician to continue professional duties as appropriate (and as considered suitable by the physician in charge of treatment), attempt to supervise as necessary, and if work has been discontinued or limited, help the physician return to appropriate work as soon as possible. The state medical society has joined with the licensing board to hire and train medical investigators who pursue complaints as well as serve as treatment monitors for physicians who have been referred to the medical board.

Often, involvement of the medical board in disciplinary or punitive action leads to requests for help. California, for example, has initiated a diversion program designed to bypass, with protection for patient safety, the time-consuming costly investigation, accusation, and hearing process in those cases of impairment in which rehabilitation and assurance of competence is in the best interest of the public and the physician. California has appointed four Diversion Evaluation Committees (each with five members, dealing with alcohol and substance abuse, physical and mental illness affecting competence) and will only accept physicians who request entry into the program. The committees review treatment facilities and designate those to which physicians may be referred. Initial referrals may be received from physicians themselves, law enforcement or judicial agencies, hospital staff, and medical and specialty societies. Files are confidential and available only to the Diversion Evaluation Committee members, who determine whether and under what conditions the physician can safely continue or resume practice. The commiteee also considers issues of confidentiality for the physician-patient and assures that the treatment and rehabilitation protocol recommended are followed. The program manager will coordinate implementation with consultation from the medical consultant.

The medical board in California also receives CII (Criminal Identification and Information) sheets from the State Department of Justice, listing physicians arrested and booked for driving while intoxicated. If a name reappears, a pattern of abuse may begin to surface, and the physician is investigated. If the investigation shows that the violation can be related to patient care, the case can proceed to filing accusation and a hearing. In other cases the physician can be warned that continuation of such conduct can lead to jeopardizing his medical license.

Patterns of potential or ongoing substance abuse can also be identified. Pharmacies may pick up self-prescribing. Since triplicate prescriptions are required for certain drugs, patterns of abuse in prescribing can be identified from a collated computer print-out. This may allow earlier intervention, limit setting, or treatment.

When there is a violation of the Medical Practice Act, by and large physicians cannot enter into voluntary programs; there is, however, great interest in exploring methods and mechanisms whereby physicians can be assisted at an early stage, and can enter the rehabilitative process prior to frank violation of the law.

REHABILITATION

It is vital to determine when a physician may safely reenter the practice of medicine. Most licensing boards prefer to proceed with probation and rehabilitation rather than impose punitive action. Probation is partially punitive, but it also allows a physician to practice in a more structured environment which minimizes risk in patient care. In some states, statutes link voluntary and nonvoluntary programs, allowing physicians to be reported to the medical board by the medical society, monitored by the medical society or other private agencies, and forgoing the necessity of filing an accusation by the board or of formally placing the physician on probation. Such programs require some sort of fail-safe method which would assure effective monitoring of the physician with periodic assessment to demonstrate that the physician was not practicing medicine beyond the limits of his capabilities. Additional mechanisms are determined for placing a physician who fails to abide by the terms of the voluntary programs into an involuntary one, and this link is an important one.

If a situation arises in which the ability of the physician to practice in the usual setting may be questioned, a period of time may be spent working in a suitable supervised environment. When treatment has been successfully completed, the committee and the physician will meet to determine employment options, goals, and objectives, in light of the physician's academic qualifications, training field or practice, physical and/or psychiatric limitations. Deficits or problems of the physician must be discussed with the prospective employer. The employer may agree to submit reports on the physician's progress at specified intervals. The physician may not leave the place of employment without notifying the committee, at which time a meeting will be held between the employee/physician and committee members to ascertain reasons for leaving and to determine the employee's performance. If performance is unsatisfactory, they will arrange needed modifications to ensure continuation of employment. If employment is terminated because of unsatisfactory performance, the committee will decide whether the physician should be returned for assessment to the contact team or some other action taken. The committee and contact team will also decide when the physician can move into a more demanding supervised environment or return to medical practice.

In addition the committee will determine whether the particular supervised practice location will be used again and obtain input from the director and other employers about their views and impressions of the work rehabilitation program.

Probations impose significant financial hardship. The Maryland Med-Chi Faculty (state medical society) has appropriated a sum of money to assist impaired physicians and help support their families if they give up practice during their rehabilitation. The money is given in interest-free loans, and monthly installments are payable beginning a year after the physician's return to practice.

Several groups have attempted to deal with family needs in other ways. Committees on outreach consisting of representatives of the auxiliary, a pharmacist, and hospital administrator provide ancillary support. These committee members can serve as an intermediary referral source as well as provide assistance to families of recovered physicians and serve as an information and education resource.

Follow-up is an important aspect of any program. In Arizona 28 physicians are currently being followed, 12 of whom were referred after July 1978. Other states use a network of activities and some ongoing contacts with patients and families. Many state societies or professional groups are sponsoring "retreats" or family growth weekends for formerly impaired physicians as well as for prevention. Inspite of the plethora of resources available, it is often difficult to begin the referral process. Concerned colleagues may feel most comfortable consulting the well-being committee of their hospital. They may contact the representative of the well-being committee of the local medical or specialty society. Most of the district branches (local psychiatric societies) of the American Psychiatric Association maintain a committee on physician well-being or the impaired physician, usually with spouse as well as professional representation. All of these committees guarantee confidentiality and anonymity while providing assistance. Ethical concerns may be voiced to local medical or specialty societies or to the State Board of Medical Examiners. Resources for affected physicians and their families include the American Medical Association Department of Mental Health and the American Psychiatric Association of Education.

In summary, local and national groups have formed in an attempt to improve case detection and treatment of impaired physicians and to help educate physicians and the public about this preventable and treatable problem. There is much potential for improvement and success with resulting savings of manpower, promoting of individual and family growth and development, and improvement of the quality of patient care.

REFERENCES

1. Scheiber SC: Emotional problems of physicians. *Ariz Med* 34:323–325, 1977.
2. AMA Council on Mental Health: The sick physician: Impairment by psychiatric disorders. *JAMA* 223:684–687, 1973.
3. Jones RE: A study of 100 physician psychiatric patients. *Am J Psychiat* 134:1119–1123, 1977.
4. Pearson MM, Strecker EA: Physicians as psychiatric patients: Private practice experience. *Am J Psychiat* 166:915–919, 1960.
5. Waring EM: Psychiatric illness in physicians: A review. *Compr Psychiat* 15:519–529, 1974.
6. Duffy JC, Litin EM: Psychiatric morbidity of physicians. *JAMA* 189:989–992, 1964.
7. *Proceedings of the Third AMA Conference on the Impaired Physician.* Chicago, AMA, 1980.
8. AMA: *Newsletter on the Impaired Physician.* Chicago, July 1979.
9. Bynder H: Physicians choose psychiatrists: Medical social structure and patterns of choice. *J Health Hum Behav* 6:83–91, 1965.

13

Residents in Family Practice
Psychosocial Support

JOLENE K. BERG and JUDITH GARRARD

Residency training, because of its intensive time and energy demands, affects many aspects of residents' lives. A survey of house staff at Stanford University School of Medicine reveals that residency training frequently has negative consequences for residents and their families. A large portion of the residents surveyed resent training demands on their families (94%), worry about relationships' ending due to training (49%), and report that they have inadequate physical exercise (68%), no time for personal reflection (59%), and worsening sex lives (49%). Furthermore, many feel powerless to influence their training experience (87%), reporting that faculty are not available to give support (53%) or to serve as advocates (49%).[1] Nelson and Henry's survey to assess the problems of family practice residents reinforces the above findings: residency frequently conflicts with residents' personal needs for leisure and socializing and with their responsibilities to spouse, children, and household.[2]

There is increasing interest in addressing problems of residents and their families, as indicated by the existence of groups such as the Humanistic Medicine Task Force (American Medical Student Association)[3] and the Committee on the Well-being of Medical Students and House Officers (Stanford University School of Medicine).[1] These groups advocate development of support systems for residents.

JOLENE K. BERG • Department of Family Practice and Community Health, St. John's Hospital, University of Minnesota Medical School, Minneapolis, Minnesota   JUDITH GARRARD • Department of Psychiatry, University of Minnesota Medical School, Minneapolis, Minnesota. Reprinted with permission from *Journal of Family Practice*, vol. 11, no. 6, 1980.

Support systems are being developed by residency programs, with examples of psychosocial support for residents described in the medical literature. Residencies in family practice utilize several methods to help residents cope with the stresses of residency training, including support groups,[4] second-year "reorientation" programs,[5] peer review committees,[6] and encounter groups.[7] In addition, residencies in specialties other than family practice report the use of retreats,[8] part-time residencies,[9] and support groups for spouses.[10]

The authors' earlier study of residency programs in six clinical specialties indicates that programs in family practice and psychiatry are more likely to offer psychosocial support to their residents than programs in internal medicine, pediatrics, surgery, or obstetrics/gynecology.[11] In order to investigate in more depth the use of psychosocial support in family practice residencies, the above study was expanded to include a larger sample of family practice programs. This chapter, which reports the results of the expanded study, has four purposes: (1) to further document the availability of 11 kinds of psychosocial support in family medicine training programs; (2) to ascertain whether program characteristics (geographic region, type of program, size of residency) influence the availability of these kinds of support; (3) to explore the different patterns of support; and (4) to examine the range of variation in frequency of night call and length of vacation.

METHODS

Instrument

From a survey of the literature and informal discussions with residents and residency program directors, the authors identified 11 kinds of psychosocial support that might be available to residents in residency training programs. The 11 kinds of support, and operational definitions of each, follow:

1. Support groups—groups of people who meet together at a scheduled time with or without a leader to discuss problems, share feelings, and give support
2. Family support groups—support groups composed of residents and their families together
3. Part-time residencies—shortening the number of residency hours per day and days per week and lengthening the duration of residency training

4. Professional counselors—psychologists, psychiatrists, or social workers available within the program to help residents with personal or family problems
5. Child-care services—day care or babysitting services sponsored by the residency program or hospital and available to residents who are parents
6. Formal "gripe sessions"—scheduled time when residents can bring complaints about the residency program before the staff
7. Seminars and/or speakers dealing with emotionally charged medical issues—for example, the dying patient, euthanasia, etc.
8. Seminars and/or speakers dealing with stresses and conflicts of being a physician—for example, physician drug abuse, balancing the professional and private life, etc.
9. Paid sick leave
10. Social activities—parties, sports events, etc., planned and sponsored by the residency program
11. Financial advisors—people to deal with income tax concerns, investments, setting up future practice, etc.

These 11 kinds of support, together with their definitions, were included on a one-page questionnaire, and respondents were asked to indicate the kinds of support available in their programs. In addition, data pertaining to frequency of night call, vacation length, and program characteristics were gathered.

Subjects

The questionnaire was mailed in 1979 with a cover letter to the directors of all family practice residency programs, as listed in the *Guide to Family Practice Residency Programs*.[12] Two follow-up mailings were used to maximize response rate. Of the 362 family practice residency programs surveyed, 96% ($N = 347$) returned completed questionnaires.

In spite of the favorable response rate, the authors wished to assess any possible differences between responding and nonresponding programs. A statistical analysis (using chi square or one-way analysis of variance, as appropriate) of three characteristics of the residency program shows that responding programs ($N = 347$) do not differ significantly from nonrespondents ($N = 15$) in terms of geographic region, size, or type of program. On this basis, one can assume that the responses are representative of all family practice residency programs and that the results are generalizable to the population as a whole.

Data Analysis

The data resulting from the survey were analyzed using different statistical methods, depending on the research question being examined. The different kinds of data and the data analysis used for each kind are described below.

Support Variables: The 11 kinds of psychosocial support (previously defined) were examined across each of three major program variables, geographic region, size, and type of program. Chi square analysis was used.

Patterns of Support: In order to explore the statistical relationships between and among the various kinds of psychosocial support, the data for all programs (N = 347) were combined. On the basis of an 11 × 11 intercorrelational matrix, the data were examined by means of factor analysis, using the normal varimax method of rotation.[13]

Night Call and Vacation: In addition to the 11 kinds of psychosocial support surveyed, two additional variables, frequency of night call and length of vacation, were each examined separately, using a three-way analysis of variance. In each of these two analyses the three independent variables were geographic region, size, and type of program.

RESULTS

Support Variables

Four geographic regions—Northeast, South, Midwest, and West (as defined in the *NIRMP Directory*[14]—are used for purposes of this study. Table I reveals that only one of the 11 kinds of psychosocial support— financial advisors—shows statistically significant differences across geographic regions. Financial advisors are less likely to be available in family practice residencies in the West (24%) than in the other three regions (52% to 55%).

A second variable, size of residency program, is defined on the basis of number of first-year residency positions available. It is felt that this accurately represents the size of the program, as 93.2% of first-year residency positions are filled.[15]

Three categories emerge: small (two to four first-year positions), medium (five to eight first-year positions), and large (nine or more first-year positions). (The authors defined size categories based on the frequency distribution of residency programs.) Table II demonstrates that six kinds of psychosocial support show statistically significant differences across size of program. For each of these six kinds of support—

Table 1. Percentage, by Geographic Region, of Residency Programs Providing Different Kinds of Psychosocial Support

	Percentage by geographic region			
Kind of psychosocial support	Northeast (N = 73)	South (N = 95)	Midwest (N = 116)	West (N = 63)
Support groups	69	57	59	59
Family support groups	23	22	19	24
Part-time residencies	20	16	15	14
Professional counselors	82	83	83	87
Child-care services	3	8	11	3
Formal gripe sessions	84	81	89	87
Seminars—medical issues	94	92	91	90
Seminars—personal and professional issues	67	73	74	73
Paid sick leave	94	92	86	92
Social activities	84	90	95	90
Financial advisors*	52	52	55	24

*$p < .001$.

Table II. Percentage, by Size of Program, of Residency Programs Providing Different Kinds of Psychosocial Support

	Percentage by size of program		
Kind of psychosocial support	Small (N = 99)	Medium (N = 179)	Large (N = 67)
Support groups**	46	67	64
Family support groups**	10	25	30
Part-time residencies***	6	17	30
Professional counselors*	76	87	90
Child-care services	8	7	8
Formal gripe sessions	83	89	81
Seminars—medical issues	89	94	92
Seminars—personal and professional issues*	65	73	82
Paid sick leave	88	93	90
Social activities*	84	94	93
Financial advisors	39	54	46

*$p < .05$.
**$p < .01$.
***$p < .001$.

support groups, family support groups, part-time residencies, professional counselors, personal/professional seminars, and social activities—small programs are less likely to offer the support than medium or large programs.

The third program variable, type of program, utilized definitions of program structure set forth by the American Academy of Family Physicians.[16] Five program types are described:

1. Community Based—program is based in a community hospital and is not affiliated with a university or medical school.
2. Community Based and University Affiliated—program is based in a community hospital, has a written contractual affiliation agreement with a university or medical school, but is administered by the hospital or other sponsoring institutions.
3. Community Based and University Administered—program is based in a community hospital, has a written contractual agreement with, and is administered by, a university or medical school.
4. University Based—program is based at, and administered by, a university or medical school.
5. Military program.

Of the 11 kinds of psychosocial support, three show statistically significant differences across type of program. Whereas both military (31%) and university-based (35%) programs are more likely to offer family support groups than the other three types of programs (13% to 20%), it is university-based programs that lead in percentage of programs offer-

Table III.   Percentage, by Type of Program, of Residency Programs Providing Different Kinds of Psychosocial Support

	Percentage by type of program				
Kind of psychosocial support	Community-based ($N=49$)	Univ-affil community-based ($N=173$)	Univ-admin community-based ($N=52$)	Univ-based ($N=57$)	Military program ($N=16$)
Support groups	55	60	56	68	69
Family support groups*	20	19	13	35	31
Part-time residencies**	20	12	15	30	0
Professional counselors	88	82	79	88	81
Child-care services	4	7	6	7	25
Formal gripe sessions*	92	88	75	77	100
Seminars—medical issues	92	91	90	95	94
Seminars—personal and professional issues	74	69	67	77	94
Paid sick leave	92	89	90	93	94
Social activities	92	88	88	96	100
Financial advisors	47	51	48	46	25

*$p < .05$.
**$p < .01$.

ing part-time residencies (30%) and military programs that lead in percentage of programs offering formal gripe sessions (100%).

Patterns of Support

In addition to examining the availability of each of the 11 kinds of support, the authors were also interested in examining patterns of support, that is, which kinds of support seem to occur together. As shown in Table IV, a factor analysis based on the 11 kinds of support included in this study results in a solution with four factors. The first factor, which reflects a psychological orientation, accounts for 60% of the variance. This first factor shows that three kinds of support—(1) seminars and/or speakers dealing with emotionally charged medical issues; (2) seminars and/or speakers dealing with stresses and conflicts of being a physician; and (3) professional counselors available in the program to help residents with personal or family problems—tend to be found together when the data are examined across all of the residency programs.

The second factor suggests a "bare bones" kind of support which consists of (1) sick leave, (2) social activities, and (3) gripe sessions. This factor accounts for 20% of the variance. Although these three kinds of support appear to be vital to any program, this combination suggests a

Table IV.   Normal Varimax Solution of Factor Analysis of 11 Kinds of Psychosocial Support

Kind of psychosocial support	"Psychological orientation" Factor 1	"Bare bones support" Factor 2	"Support group orientation" Factor 3	"Family orientation" Factor 4	Communality
Support groups	.1552	.1751	.5600	.0873	.3759
Family support groups	.0402	.0802	.6150	.1390	.4056
Part-time residencies	.0979	−.0165	.0661	.1310	.0314
Professional counselors	.4610	.1620	.0751	.1174	.2582
Child-care services	.0162	.0822	.0658	.4194	.1872
Formal gripe sessions	.2320	.3874	.0730	.0543	.2122
Seminars—medical issues	.5818	.2914	.0079	.1314	.4408
Seminars—personal and professional issues	.5492	.1166	.1271	.0710	.3364
Paid sick leave	.0694	.4972	.0872	.0688	.2644
Social activities	.1524	.4101	.0885	.0882	.2070
Financial advisors	.1170	.1092	.0529	.4342	.2169
Amounts of variance accounted for	60%	20%	10%	10%	—

minimum level of support that is probably least taxing of the faculty's time and personal investment in the resident as a person.

The third factor, reflecting a support-group orientation, consists of two items: (1) support groups for residents, and (2) family support groups.

The final factor indicates a family orientation and consists of three items: (1) financial advisors, (2) child care, and (3) part-time residencies. This factor also accounts for ten percent of the variance. As the results in the preceding section indicate, few residency programs offer child care or part-time residencies, but in those programs in which these are options, they tend to be found together and with the additional availability of a financial advisor.

Night Call and Vacation

Because vacation and evenings away from work help to relieve the time pressures of residency training, length of vacation and frequency of night call (both for first-year residents) are assessed, as shown in Tables V and VI. On the average, first-year residents cover night call every 3.64 nights. Across each of the three program variables—geographic region, size, and type of program—frequency of night call does not vary significantly when the remaining two variables are held constant. On the other hand length of paid vacation does show statistically significant differences by geographic region and by type of program. Controlling for the remaining two variables, one finds that on the average residency programs in the Northeast and West offer longer vacations (2.62 weeks and 2.71 weeks) than do southern (2.21 weeks) or midwestern (2.25 weeks) programs (p < .001). In the same fashion, controlling for geographic region and size of program, one sees that university-based programs offer longer vacations (2.61 weeks) than do the other four

Table V. Frequency of First-year Night Call
in Family Practice Residency Programs

Night call interval every (no.) night	Number and percent of residency programs	
	Number	Percent
2–2.9	2	<1
3–3.9	179	52
4–4.9	138	40
5–5.9	19	5
6–6.9	3	1
7–7.9	3	1
No night call	2	<1

Table VI. Length of First-year Paid Vacation in Family Practice Residency Programs

Number of vacation weeks	Number and percent of residency programs	
	Number	Percent
1	3	1
2	234	68
3	74	21
4	35	10

types of programs (2.25 to 2.41 weeks). This latter difference is statistically significant at the $p < .05$ level.

DISCUSSION

On a national basis, there is considerable similarity among family practice residency programs in terms of the kinds of psychosocial support offered to residents. This similarity may be related to the fact that family practice residency programs have developed over a short time span under well-defined guidelines.

Size of residency program, however, is a factor in the amount of formal support offered to residents. It is not surprising that small programs are generally less likely than larger programs to offer the kinds of support surveyed. It may not be cost-effective to provide numerous formal kinds of support to a small group of residents. More important, in small programs there is likely to be closer interaction between and among residents and faculty, thus providing valuable informal support systems and reducing the need for the more structured kinds of support examined in this survey.

In general, family practice residency programs offer considerable psychosocial support to their residents. Several factors may play a role in this circumstance. First, family practice faculty are frequently drawn away from private practice into academia because it allows for a more flexible lifestyle and more time for personal and family needs. This faculty background might make family practice teachers more sensititve to the needs of their residents. Furthermore, family practice as a specialty emphasizes preventive, holistic health care. It is possible that this orientation has been incorporated into the structure of family practice residency programs, with residency programs showing concern for the resident as a "total person."

On the other hand, of the 11 kinds of support surveyed, those which are most supportive of the resident's family needs—family support groups, part-time residencies, and child-care services—are least likely to be offered. Although residency programs as a whole rarely offer child-care services, family practice programs lag behind programs in other specialities (obstetrics/gynecology, pediatrics, psychiatry, and internal medicine) in the frequency with which part-time residencies are available.[11] Since family responsibilities are frequently a major source of conflict for the resident, family practice residencies should consider incorporating into their programs more support options related to family needs in addition to the support already available that addresses the residents' individual needs. By providing support of both individual and family needs of residents, family practice residency programs will exemplify the field's commitment to the whole person within the context of environment, community, and family.[17]

REFERENCES

1. Weinstein H, Blumenthal S: The human costs of medical education: A study of medical students, house officers, and their partners. Paper presented at Association for Academic Psychiatry annual meeting, San Antonio, Tex, March, 1980.
2. Nelson EG, Henry WF: Psychosocial factors seen as problems by family practice residents and their spouses. *J Fam Pract* 6:581, 1978.
3. Taylor C: The humanistic medicine task force. *Annu Conf Med Educ* 18:358, 1979.
4. Kantner TR, Vastyan EA: Coping with stress in family practice residency training. *J Fam Pract* 7:599, 1978.
5. Rhyne RL Jr, Magill MK, Selig CF, et al.: A reorientation program for second year residents. *Fam Med Teacher* 12:10, 1980.
6. Engebretsen B: Peer review in graduate education. *N Engl J Med* 296:1230, 1977.
7. Johnson AH: Resident self-awareness through group process. *J Fam Pract* 4:681, 1977.
8. Bergman AB, Rothenberg MB, Telzrow RW: A "retreat" for pediatric interns. *Pediatrics* 64:528, 1979.
9. Kaplan HI: Part-time residency training: An approach to the graduate training of some women physicians. *JAMWA* 27:648, 1972.
10. Bergman AS: Marital stress and medical training: An experience with a support group for medical house staff wives. *Pediatrics* 65:944, 1980.
11. Berg JK, Garrard J: Psychosocial support in residency training programs. *J Med Educ* 55:851, 1980.
12. *Guide to Family Practice Residency Programs.* American Academy of Family Physicians and American Medical Student Association, 1979.
13. Harman HH: *Modern Factor Analysis.* Chicago, University of Chicago Press, 1967.
14. *NIRMP Directory.* Evanston, Ill, National Intern and Resident Matching Program, 1979.
15. Annual survey of family practice residency programs (AAFP Reprint #150). Kansas City, Mo, American Academy of Family Physicians, 1980.
16. Approved graduate residency training programs in family practice (AAFP Reprint #135B). Kansas City, Mo, American Academy of Family Physicians, 1980.
17. Meeting the challenge of family practice. The report of the ad hoc committee on education for family practice of the Council on Medical Education. Chicago, AMA, 1966, pp 7–8.

VI

Recommendations

14

Conclusions and Recommendations

STEPHEN C. SCHEIBER and BRIAN B. DOYLE

This book introduces the reader to a variety of problems associated with the impaired physician. In this final section we would like to summarize briefly the recommendations which have emerged for further action. The recommendations include those applying to medical students, those to house officers, those to practicing physicians, and those to all three of these groups. In addition, the authors have recommended studies which would improve prevention and treatment efforts for the impaired physician.

First are several recommendations applying to medical students. Admissions committees should play an expanded role by acquiring more comprehensive health data on applicants to medical school, and by screening out candidates for drug addiction, alcoholism, and other psychiatric disorders. Once admitted to medical school, students who are identified as high risk should have a special support system available. The period of orientation to medical school provides an excellent opportunity to develop trust and cooperation among students, faculty, and administration; it is also a good time for students to learn about primary prevention. Another important time is the transition in medical school from the preclinical to clinical years. Levels of student interest and anxiety are high, so there are good chances to learn more about preventing impairment and managing the stresses of clinical life.

There need to be more women faculty members available as role models for medical students, not just as teachers and supervisors, but as consultants and sources of help. The dean of student affairs can appropriately expand on the leadership role in the medical school concerning prevention by addressing issues of student stress and impairment and

STEPHEN C. SCHEIBER ● Department of Psychiatry, University of Arizona College of Medicine, Tucson, Arizona   BRIAN B. DOYLE ● Department of Psychiatry and Behavioral Sciences, George Washington University School of Medicine and Health Sciences, Washington, D.C.

keeping these prominent at faculty and administration discussions. The deans and others, notably in departments of psychiatry and the primary-care disciplines, should encourage small groups made up of students, faculty, and administrators. Such groups can have relief of stress and prevention of impairment as primary or as indirect goals. In addition to the established academic counseling for students with study habit difficulties, medical schools need to establish ways to identify and help those with nonacademic troubles. Services made available to students having sexual difficulties may prove particularly useful.

The recommendations for house officers as a group, while few, are more ambitious. These include decreasing work overload and fatigue and providing part-time residencies, particularly (but not exclusively) for women. Residency directors can attend to improving the quality of life by attention to numerous support systems issues, such as making it possible for families to get together with house officers during mealtimes and evenings when on call. Psychological support, adequate vacations, and encouragement of resident groups would also be helpful.

For the practicing physician, there are a variety of recommendations. Organized medicine can increase existing responsibilities for physician impairment, especially in the areas of alcohol and drug abuse. Developing measurable objectives to reduce incidence and prevalence, especially of problems related to alcohol and other drugs, would be useful. There need to be ongoing efforts to encourage physicians to recognize signs and symptoms of personal difficulty and to seek help. Continuing Medical Education activities should include materials and approaches relating to issues of physician impairment. Psychiatrists have developed Continuing Medical Education credits for small study groups which have peer supervision and learning as a direct agenda. Other medical specialties could consider this model, which clearly has potential for relieving physician stress as well as increasing knowledge. For all physicians there needs to be easy access to treatment, with attention to privacy, confidentiality, trust, and sensitivity.

There are special roles for psychiatrists in relation to the impaired physician. Psychiatrists need to improve their expertise in treating physician-patients. More psychiatrists should collaborate with colleagues in other medical disciplines to identify and treat alcohol and other drug abuse. Finally, psychiatrists need to attend to the factors within their own discipline which contribute to the current impression of a higher than usual suicide rate in that specialty.

There are some recommendations which apply to medical students, house officers, and practicing physicians alike. With all three groups, educators and administrators need to take more initiative and concerted actions, not simply about abuse of alcohol and other drugs, but also about the stresses which contribute to the other syndromes of physician impairment. There is a clear need for more educational experiences at all levels of medical education to increase the knowledge base about impairment, and even more important, to increase the willingness of persons in medicine to seek help. For all, more support groups are indicated for primary prevention, to ease stress, and for greater self-awareness. Women students and physicians may well profit particularly from support groups and support networks. Similarly, the families and spouses of people in medicine would benefit from support groups. At all levels in medicine, current efforts at early detection and rapid treatment need bolstering. The recent proliferation of state medical society networks for the impaired physician is heartening, but more work on the local level is necessary. In the tragic situation of suicide, the concept of "postvention" deserves further implementation. Families and colleagues need to express their feelings about the suicide. The medical community can usefully investigate what led to this final act with a view to prevention. Such "postvention" is appropriate in the medical school, residency program, or local medical community.

In addition to practical recommendations, a number of suggestions for further study have also emerged. Most simply, we need better epidemiological data on impaired physicians generally; specifically, more data are required on psychiatric hospitalization of medical students and physicians. Further studies on alcohol-related problems in medical students would be helpful, especially if they resulted in clearer criteria of abuse. These could be increasingly important because of current concern about increasing amounts of drinking among adolescents and young adults generally.

Our current methods of treatment, while well intentioned and variably successful, suffer from being nonspecific. Controlled studies are necessary to define which type of therapy is best for which physician-patients.

Recent years have seen a heartening trend in increased attention to the problems of the impaired physician. In this book we have focused on these, not just because medical students and physicians are an important group of professional persons, but also because they are the special interest of the contributing authors, nearly all of whom are substantially involved in psychiatric education. We hope that our observations and suggestions will be helpful to medical professional persons and their families, medical educators and administrators. We believe that other persons will find that this work applies outside medicine as well. There are many groups of persons who do stressful, important, and rewarding work; other medical and mental health professionals, the clergy, law enforcement personnel, dentists, business executives, politicians, persons in the media are just a few. We in medicine strongly want and need to care "for our own." Surely others feel similarly about their colleagues and friends. In this book we hope to give specific forms to the general wish to care for and about our fellows. The needs are pressing, and the rewards of intervention are great when successful. We want to provide effective care for our patients. Clearly, to do so, we must provide effective care for ourselves and for each other.

Appendix A

State Medical Society/Specialty Society Programs to Aid Impaired Physicians

Emanuel M. Steindler, Director of the Department of Mental Health of the American Medical Association, has kindly given permission to print a listing of the State Medical Society/Specialty Society Programs to aid impaired physicians, along with the names of medical society staff contacts.

State Medical Society/Specialty Society
Programs to Aid Impaired Physicians

State programs	Committee chairperson	Staff contact
Alabama—Impaired Physician Committee; combined voluntary and coercive program. Components: prevention, case-finding, intervention, treatment referral Hotline: (205) 263-3947	Charles Herlihy, M.D. Suite 510 840 Montclair Rd. Birmingham AL 35213 (205-591-3451)	George E. Oetting, Ed.D. Director of Education Medical Association of the State of Alabama 19 S. Jackson St. P.O. Box 1900-C Montgomery AL 36104 (205-263-6641)
Alaska—Established "Friends of Medicine" program in 1981.	Randolph M. Hall, M.D. 4045 Lake Otis Parkway Anchorage AK 99504 (907-274-7543)	Martha MacDermaid Administrative Secretary Alaska State Medical Assn. 1135 W. 8th Ave. Anchorage AK 99501 (907-277-6891)
Arizona—Physician's Health Committee; combined voluntary and coercive program. Components: case-finding, intervention, treatment referral, after-care monitoring, re-entry	Thomas E. Bittker, M.D. Arizona Health Plan P.O. Box 5000 Phoenix AZ 85010 (602-257-8800)	Bruce E. Robinson, M.D. Executive Director Arizona Medical Assn. 810 W. Bethany Home Rd. Phoenix AZ 85013 (602-246-8901)
Arkansas—No formal program (The Society makes nominations for the state medical board which handles all referrals concerning impaired physicians).	——	Clifton C. Long, M.D. Executive Vice-President Arkansas Medical Society 214 N. 12th St., Box 1208 Fort Smith AR 72902 (501-782-8218)

Gail B. Jara
California Medical Assn.
731 Market St.
San Francisco CA 94103
(415-777-2000)

Donald Taugher, M.D.
58 Via Castanada
Monterey CA 93940

California—Committee on the Well-Being of Physicians; strictly voluntary program.
Components: prevention, intervention, treatment referral, financial assistance
Hotline: (415) 756-7787 (Northern California); (213) 383-2691 (Southern California)

Brian K. Stutheit
Colorado Medical Society
1601 E. 19th Ave.
Denver CO 80218
(303-861-1221)

John Avery, M.D.
2750 Broadway
Boulder CO 80302

Colorado—Committee on Health and Rehabilitation; combined voluntary and coercive program.
Components: case-finding, intervention, treatment referral, after-care monitoring, re-entry

Timothy B. Norbeck
Executive Director
Connecticut State Medical Society
160 St. Ronan Terr.
New Haven CT 06511
(203-865-0587)

Duncan R. MacMaster, M.D.
Main Street
Southbury CT 06488

Connecticut—Currently in development

Anne Shane Bader
Medical Society of Delaware
1925 Lovering Ave.
Wilmington DE 19806

Calvin B. Hearne, M.D.
1805 Foulk Rd.
Wilmington DE 19810

Delaware—Impaired Physician's Committee; combined voluntary and coercive program.
Components: case-finding, intervention, treatment referral, after-care monitoring, re-entry, financial assistance

Francisco P. Ferraraccio
Medical Society of District of Columbia
2007 Eye St. NW
Washington DC 20006
(202-223-2230)

Clifton Gruver, M.D.
1145 19th St. NW, #202
Washington DC 20036
(202-452-8020)

District of Columbia—Committee on the Impaired Physician

Florida—Committee on Impaired Physicians; combined voluntary and coercive program.
Components: case-finding, intervention, treatment referral, after-care monitoring, re-entry, financial assistance
Hotline: (305) 667-8717

Chairman: Guy T. Selander, M.D.
1736 University Park Blvd.
Jacksonville FL 32216
(904-725-0200)

Medical Director: Delores A. Morgan, M.D.
7400 S.W. 62nd Avenue
Miami FL 33143

Edward D. Hagan
Director, Scientific Activities
Florida Medical Foundation
760 Riverside Avenue
P.O. Box 2411
Jacksonville FL 33203

Georgia—Disabled Doctors Committee/ Physicians Consultant Committee; combined voluntary and coercive program.
Components: prevention, case-finding, intervention, treatment referral, after-care monitoring, re-entry, financial assistance

Spencer G. Mullins, M.D.
105 Campbell Hill St.
Marietta GA 30060

G. Douglas Talbott, M.D.
Ridgeview Institute
3995 South Cobb Dr.
Smyrna GA 30081
(404-435-2570)

J. Tom Sawyer
Medical Association of Georgia
938 Peachtree St. NW
Atlanta GA 30309
(404-876-7535)

Hawaii—Physician's Committee (Subcommittee of the Peer Review Committee)/ Honolulu County Medical Society (90% of Hawaii physicians); combined voluntary and coercive program.

Alan B. Hawk, M.D.
Straub Clinic and Hospital
888 S. King
Honolulu HI 96813

Bess Chang
Honolulu County Medical Society
320 Ward Ave.
Honolulu HI 96813
(908-536-6988)

Idaho—Currently in development.

Donald W. Sower
Idaho Medical Assn.
407 W. Bannock St.
Boise ID 83701
(208-344-7888)

Illinois—Panel for the Impaired Physician; combined voluntary and coercive program.
Components: case-finding, intervention, treatment referral, financial assistance

Lee Gladstone, M.D.
320 E. Huron
Chicago IL 60611

Larry Boress, Director
Division of Medical Services
Illinois State Medical Society
55 E. Monroe, Suite 3510
Chicago IL 60603
(312-782-1654)

Indiana—Commission on Physician Impairment; combined voluntary and coercive program.
Components: prevention, case-finding, intervention, treatment referral, after-care monitoring, re-entry
Hotline: (800) 382-1721 (Indiana only); recorded messages after hours

Richard Campbell, M.D.
3625 E. 71st St.
Indianapolis IN 46220

Sara Kline, R.N.
Indiana State Medical Society
3935 N. Meridian
Indianapolis IN 46208
(317-925-7545)

Iowa—Committee on Assistance Program for Troubled Physicians; combined voluntary and coercive program.
Components: prevention, case-finding, intervention, treatment referral, after-care monitoring

Hormoz Rassekh, M.D.
201 Ridge St.
Council Bluffs IA 51501
(712-328-1858)

Tina Prettakes
Iowa Medical Society
1001 Grand Ave.
West Des Moines IA 50265
(515-223-1401)

Kansas—Impaired Physician Program; combined voluntary and coercive program.
Components: prevention, case-finding, intervention, treatment referral, financial assistance

Ivan E. Rhodes, M.D.
3333 E. Central
Wichita KS 67208
(316-685-1291)

Val Braun
Kansas Medical Society
1300 Topeka Blvd.
Topeka KS 66612
(913-235-2383)

Kentucky—Committee on Impaired Physicians; combined voluntary and coercive program.
Components: case-finding, treatment referral, after-care monitoring

David L. Stewart, M.D.
Suite 214
Professional Park
2120 Newburg Rd.
Louisville KY 40205

Robert E. Klinglesmith
Kentucky Medical Assn.
3532 Ephraim McDowell Dr.
Louisville KY 40205
(502-459-9790)

James H. Stewart, M.D.
Louisiana State Medical Society
1700 Josephine St.
New Orleans   LA   70113
(504-561-1033)

Gene L. Usdin, M.D.
1522 Aline St.
New Orleans   LA   70115

Louisiana—Committee on the Impaired Physician

Frank O. Stred
Maine Medical Assn.
524 Western Ave.
Augusta   ME   04338

Robert M. Knowles, M.D.
52 Gilman St.
Portland   ME   04101

Maine—Physicians Concerned Committee; coercive program (physicians reported as required by law)
Components: case-finding, intervention, treatment referral, after-care monitoring

Constance Townsend
Medical and Chirurgical Faculty of Maryland
1211 Cathedral St.
Baltimore   MD   21201
(301-539-0872)

Joseph Chambers, M.D.
4001 Glenrose St.
Kensington   MD   20795
(301-949-1722)

Maryland—Committee on Physician Rehabilitation; combined voluntary and coercive program.
Components: case-finding, intervention, treatment referral, after-care monitoring, financial assistance
24-hour Hotline: (301) 467-4224

Fran G. Broecker
Massachusetts Medical Society
22 The Fenway
Boston   MA   02215
(617-536-8812)

Richard Curran, M.D.
Salem Hospital
Salem   MA   01907

Massachusetts—Committee on the Disabled Physician; combined voluntary and coercive program.

Marcelyn Ireland
Michigan State Medical Society
P.O. Box 950
120 W. Saginaw
East Lansing   MI   48823
(517-337-1351)

John R. Ylvisaker, M.D.
875 Canterbury Crescent
Bloomfield Hills   MI   48013

Michigan—Program to Assist Impaired Physicians; strictly voluntary program.
Components: prevention, case-finding, intervention, treatment referral, after-care monitoring, re-entry, financial assistance

Minnesota—Committee on the Impaired Physician

Thomas G. Briggs, M.D.
3220 Bellaire
White Bear Lake MN 55110

Donald Linder
Minnesota Medical Assn.
Health Associations Center
Suite 400, 2221 University Ave. SE
Minneapolis MN 55414
(612-378-1875)

Mississippi—Physicians Consultant Committee; combined voluntary and coercive program.
Components: case-finding, intervention, in-patient/out-patient treatment, two-year after-care therapeutic program (after-care and re-entry monitoring), re-education, financial assistance
Hotline: (800) 682-6415

Doyle P. Smith, M.D.
Suite 103, Medical Plaza
2969 University Drive
Jackson, MS 39216

Charles L. Mathews
Mississippi State Medical Assn.
735 Riverside Dr.
P.O. Box 5229
Jackson MS 39216
(601-356-5433)

Missouri—Committee on the Impaired Physician; combined voluntary and coercive program.
Components: case-finding, intervention, treatment referral, after-care monitoring, re-entry

Donald E. McIntosh, M.D.
142 Research Medical Office Bldg.
6400 Prospect
Kansas City MO 64132
(816-444-1139)

Michael Porter
Missouri State Medical Assn.
P.O. Box 1028
Jefferson City MO 65102
(314-636-5151)

Montana—Special Committee on Health and Well-Being of Physicians; combined voluntary and coercive program.
Components: intervention, treatment referral

Duncan D. Burford, M.D.
1116 N. 29th St.
Billings MT 59101

G. Brian Zins
Montana Medical Assn.
2021 11th Ave., Suite 12
Helena MT 59601
(406-443-4000)

Nebraska—Ad-Hoc Committee on the Impaired Physician.

James E. Kelsey, M.D.
100 S. 19th St.
Room 135
Omaha NE 68102

Kenneth Neff
Nebraska Medical Assn.
1512 1st National Bank Bldg.
Lincoln NE 68508
(402-474-4472)

John N. Chappell, M.D.
Professor of Psychiatry
University of Nevada–Reno
Anderson Medical Sciences Bldg.
Reno NV 89557
(702-784-4917)

Kathy Nigro
Nevada State Medical Assn.
3660 Baker Lane
Reno NV 89509
(702-825-6788)

Nevada—Physicians Aid Committee; strictly voluntary program.
Components: prevention, case-finding, intervention, treatment referral, after-care monitoring, re-entry, financial assistance

Robert J. Chapman, M.D.
Hitchcock Clinic
Hanover NH 03755

Hamilton S. Putnam
New Hampshire Medical Society
4 Park St.
Concord NH 03301
(603-224-1909)

New Hampshire—Physician Effectiveness Section; strictly voluntary program.
Components: prevention programs, case-finding, intervention, treatment referral, after-care monitoring, re-entry, financial assistance

Edward T. Carden, M.D.
W. 3rd and Church St.
Morrestown NJ 08057

Lynda Dorsey
Medical Society of New Jersey
2 Princess Road
Lawrenceville NJ 08648
(609) 896-1766

New Jersey—Impaired Physicians Committee; combined voluntary and coercive program.
Hotline: (609) 896-1884

James L. Pollock, Jr., M.D.
Fort Bayard Medical Center
P.O. Box 219
Fort Bayard NM 88036
(505-537-3189)

Ralph Marshall
New Mexico Medical Society
2650 Yale Blvd. SE
Albuquerque NM 87106
(505-247-0539)

New Mexico—Physicians Aid Committee; strictly voluntary program.
Components: case-finding, intervention, treatment referral

Brian R. Nagy, M.D.
Elmira Medical Arts Center
Elmira NY 14901

Henry I. Fineberg, M.D.
Medical Society of State of New York
420 Lakeville Rd.
Lake Success NY 11042
(516-488-6100)

New York—Physician's Committee; strictly voluntary program.
Components: case-finding, intervention, treatment referral, after-care monitoring

North Carolina—Committee on Physician Health and Effectiveness; strictly voluntary program (when voluntary efforts fail, the referring party is instructed to contact the licensing/disciplinary board directly).

Theodore R. Clark, M.D.
P.O. Box 1569
Pinehurst NC 28374

William N. Hilliard
North Carolina Medical Society
222 N. Person St.
P.O. Box 27167
Raleigh NC 27611
(918-833-3836)

North Dakota—Impaired Physicians Committee; combined voluntary and coercive program.
Components: prevention, case-finding, intervention, treatment referral

A. E. Samuelson, M.D.
P.O. Box 1975
Bismarck ND 58502

David J. Peske
North Dakota Medical Association
Assistant Executive Vice President
P.O. 498
810 E. Rosser
Bismarck ND 58502
(701-223-9475)

Ohio—Subcommittee on Impaired Physicians; combined voluntary and coercive program.
Components: prevention, case-finding, intervention, treatment referral

Perry R. Ayres, M.D.
Harding Hospital
445 E. Granville Rd.
Worthington OH 43085
(614-885-5381)

Robert Clinger
Ohio State Medical Assn.
600 S. High St.
Columbus OH 43215
(614-228-6971)

Oklahoma—Physicians' Care Committee; combined voluntary and coercive program.

Joseph B. Ruffin, M.D.
400 NW 16th St.
Oklahoma City OK 73104
(405-524-0909)

Lyle Kelsey
Oklahoma State Medical Assn.
601 NW Expressway
Oklahoma City OK 73118
(405-843-9571)

Oregon—Physicians' Committee; combined voluntary and coercive program.
Components: prevention, case-finding, intervention, treatment referral, re-entry

Kent Neff, M.D.
9205 SW Barnes Rd.
Portland OR 97225

James A. Kronenberg
Oregon Medical Assn.
5210 SW Corbett St.
Portland OR 97201
(503-226-1555)

Donna Wenger
Pennsylvania Medical Society
P.O. Box 301
20 Erford Rd.
Lemoyne   PA   17043
(717-763-7151)

Howard E. Lawton
Rhode Island Medical Society
106 Francis St.
Providence   RI   02903
(401-331-3208)

Charles Johnson
South Carolina Medical Assn.
3325 Medical Park Rd.
P.O. Box 11188
Columbia   SC   29211
(803-252-6311)

Jan Anderson
South Dakota State Medical Assn.
608 West Ave. North
Sioux Falls   SD   57104
(605-336-1965)

Abraham J. Twerski, M.D.
St. Francis General Hospital
45th Street off Penn Avenue
Pittsburgh   PA   15201

Herbert Rakatansky, M.D.
Moshassuck Medical Center
Suite 305
1 Randall Square
Providence   RI   02904
(401-726-3450)

S. Hunter Rentz, M.D.
1701 St. Julian Pl.
Columbia   SC   29204
(803-254-3386)

Coordinators:
T. H. Sattler, M.D.
Yankton Clinic
Yankton   SD   57078
C. E. Tesar, M.D.
2001 7th
Rapid City   SD   55701

Pennsylvania—Committee on the Impaired Physician; strictly voluntary program. Components: prevention, case-finding, intervention, treatment referral, after-care monitoring

Rhode Island—Impaired Physicians Committee; combined voluntary and coercive program.

South Carolina—Committee on Alcohol, Drug Abuse and Impaired Physicians; combined voluntary and coercive program. Components: case-finding, intervention, treatment referral, after-care monitoring, re-entry

South Dakota—Physician Rehabilitation Committee; combined voluntary and coercive program. Components: intervention, treatment referral

Tennessee—Impaired Physician Committee; combined voluntary and coercive program.
Components: case-finding, intervention, treatment referral, after-care monitoring, re-entry, financial assistance, formal re-education clerkship
Hotline: (615) 327-2711 (outside Nashville, call collect)

John B. Dorian, M.D.
3262 Millington Rd.
Memphis TN 38127

Don Alexander
Tennessee Medical Assn.
112 Louise Ave.
Nashville TN 37203
(615-327-1541)

Texas—Committee on Physician Health and Rehabilitation; combined voluntary and coercive program.
Components: intervention, treatment referral, re-entry

Percy E. Lowe, M.D.
902 Frostwood #179
Houston TX 77024

Barbara Provine
Texas Medical Assn.
1801 N. Lamar Blvd.
Austin TX 78701
(512-477-6704)

Utah—Physicians Committee; strictly voluntary program.
Components: case-finding, intervention, treatment referral, re-entry

Bryce J. Fairbanks, M.D.
34 S. 5th St. East
Suite 207
Salt Lake City UT 84102

Hoyt W. Brewster
Utah State Medical Assn.
540 E. 5th St. South
Salt Lake City UT 84102
(801-355-7477)

Vermont—Impaired Physician Committee established in 1980.

William Beach, M.D.
Brattleboro Retreat
Brattleboro VT 05301

D. Robert Vautier
Vermont State Medical Society
136 Main St.
Montpelier VT 05602
(802-223-7898)

Virginia—Physicians Health and Effectiveness Committee; combined voluntary and coercive program.

William H. Barney, M.D.
1935 Thomson Drive
Lynchburg VA 24501

William C. Osburn
Medical Society of Virginia
4205 Dover Rd.
Richmond VA 23221
(804-353-2721)

Washington—Committee on Personal Problems of Physicians; strictly voluntary program.
Hotline: (800) 552-7237

Marcelle F. Dunning, M.D.
1120 Cherry St.
Seattle WA 98104

Richard Gorman
Washington State Medical Assn.
2033 Sixth Ave.
Seattle WA 98121
(206-623-4801)

West Virginia—Committee on Physician Services; coercive program.
Components: prevention, intervention, treatment referral, (still in developmental phase)

William N. Walker, Jr., M.D.
Route 2, Box 36
Bridgeport WV 26330

Charles R. Lewis
West Virginia State Medical Assn.
1526 Charleston National Plaza
P.O. Box 1031
Charleston WV 25324
(304-346-0551)

Wisconsin—Impaired Physician Program established 1977. Combined voluntary/coercive program, although referral to board is not necessarily automatic.

Gerald C. Kempthorne, M.D.
P.O. Box 466
Spring Green WI 53588

John C. LaBissonier
State Medical Society of Wisconsin
330 E. Lakeside St.
P.O. Box 1109
Madison WI 53701
(608-257-6781)

Wyoming—Committee on Impaired Physicians; combined voluntary and coercive program.
Components: intervention, treatment referral, re-entry

Roger A. Brown
Wyoming Medical Society
1920 Evans Ave.
P.O. Drawer 4009
Cheyenne WY 82001
(307-635-2424)

Specialty society programs

American Academy of Family Physicians
Committee on Mental Health

Chairman:
Donald M. Keith, M.D.
17191 Bothell Way NE
Seattle WA 98155
(206-364-8250)

Alan Woodall
American Academy of Family Physicians
1740 W. 92nd St.
Kansas City MO 64114
(816-333-9700)

American College of Obstetricians and
Gynecologists

———

Shirley Shelton
American College of Obstetricians and
Gynecologists
1 E. Wacker Dr.
Suite 2700
Chicago IL 60601 (312-222-1600)

American Occupational Medical Association

Chairperson:
Fern Asma, M.D.
Illinois Bell Telephone Co.
HQ 14-F
212 W. Washington St.
Chicago IL 60606

———

American Psychiatric Association, Committee on the Impaired Physician

Chairperson:
Robert E. Jones, M.D.
1025 Walnut St.
Philadelphia PA
(215-922-6695)

Carolyn B. Robinowitz, M.D.
American Psychiatric Assn.
1700 18th St. NW
Washington DC 20009
(202-797-4900)

Appendix B

Bibliography on the Impaired Physician

Emanuel M. Steindler, Director of the Department of Mental Health of the American Medical Association, has kindly given permission to print the bibliography on the impaired physician prepared by the American Medical Association.

Bibliography on the Impaired Physician

I. Disabled Doctors Programs

AMA Council on Mental Health: The sick physician (impairment by psychiatric disorders, including alcoholism and drug dependence). *JAMA* 223(6):684–687, 1973.

APTP means help. *J Iowa Med Soc* 70(7):318, 1980.

Ashton MM Sr: Motivating the disabled doctor: A hospital program. April 1975. Available from the AMA Dept. of Mental Health

Bates RC: Physicians heal thy colleagues. *Mich Med* 78(29):530, 1979.

Berman JI, Sargeant J: Organized medicine and the drug-abusing physician. *Maryland State Med J* 23:37–42, 1974.

Breiner SJ: The impaired physician. *Bull—Oakland Co Med Soc* 53(2):9–10, 1979.

Breiner SJ: A position statement of OCMS impaired physician committee. *Bull—Oakland Co Med Soc* 53(10):11, 1979.

Bittker TE: The distressed physician: Where do we go from here? *Ariz Med* 35(7):469–472, 1978.

Clinger RD: Help for the alcoholic physician in Ohio. *Alc: Clin Exp Res* 1(2):139–141, 1977.

Gold N: Doctors get sick, too. *Aust Fam Phys* 9(5):337–342, 1980.

Green RC Jr, Carroll GJ, Buxton WD: *The Care and Management of the Sick and Incompetent Physician.* Springfield, Ill, Charles C Thomas, 1978.

Henry S: Alcohol and drugs: The doctor's own prescription (Canadian impaired physician programs). *Can Med Assoc J* 120(87):989–996, 1979.

Hugunin MB: Helping the Impaired Physician. *Proceedings of the AMA Conference on "The Impaired Physician: Answering the Challenge,"* Feb. 4–6, 1977. American Medical Assoc., 535 N. Dearborn St., Chicago IL 60610.

Hurting Inside: A Special Issue on the Impaired Physician. *LACMA Phys Bull Los Angeles Co Med Soc* 110(1):31–49, 1980.

Impaired physicians now may find help through MSMS program. *Mich Med* July 1975, p 413.

The impaired physician. *Texas Med* 73:105–108, 1977.

Impaired physicians: Medicine bites the bullet. *Med World News,* July 24, 1978, p. 40.

Johnston PP: The impaired physician: A treatable problem. *J Indiana Med Assoc* 71(11):1058–1060, 1978.

Kempthorne GC: The impaired physician—the role of the state medical society. *Wis Med J* 78:24–25, 1979.

Korcok M: Impaired doctor programs growing. *Focus Alc Drug Issues* 3(2):16–18, 1980.

KMS impaired physician program: Statement of purpose. *J Kans Med Soc* 79(8):372–375, 1978.

Ludlam JE: Physician rehabilitation: A better alternative to punishment. *Hosp Med Staff* 5(4):8–11, 1976.

McGuire M: The panel for the impaired physician. *Ill Med J* 151(4):286–291, 1977.

New help for disabled physicians. *Ohio State Med J* 71:641–644, 1975.

New MSMA statewide program offers assistance to the impaired physician. *Missouri Med* 76(2):95–96, 1979.

Physicians' committee. *N Y State J Med* 75:420–423, 1975.

Rassekh H: A program for the impaired physician. *J Iowa Med Soc* 68(3):81–84, 1978.

Robertson JJ: The impaired physician. *Proceedings of the Third AMA Conference on the Impaired Physician, Sept. 29–Oct. 1, 1978.* American Medical Assoc., 535 N. Dearborn Street, Chicago   IL   60610.

Rosenberg CL: Doctor rehabilitation: It is working. *Med Economics* Nov. 26, 1979, p 115.

Sargent DA: Helping troubled colleagues. *J Tenn Med Assoc* 72(7):497–498, 1979.

Scheiber SC: A comprehensive statewide approach to the sick doctor *Ariz Med* 32(12):933–935, 1975.

Scheiber SC: Emotional problems of physicians: II. Current approaches to the problem. *Ariz Med* 35(5):336–337, 1978.

Smith RF: Committee on impaired physicians breaks conspiracy of denial. *Mich Med* 78(29):527–528, 1979.

Statewide impaired physician program created. *Wis Med J* 79(7):42, 1980.

Steindler EM: *The Impaired Physician—An Interpretative Summary of the AMA Conference on "The Disabled Doctor: Challenge to the Profession," April 11–12, 1975.* American Medical Assoc., 535 N. Dearborn Street, Chicago   IL   60610.

Talbott GD: The disabled doctors' program of Georgia. *Alc: Clin Exp Res* 1(2):143–146, 1977.

Talbott GD, Holderfield H, Shoemaker KE, et al: The disabled doctors' plan for Georgia. *J Med Assoc Georgia* 65(3):71–76, 1976.

Talbott GD, Richardson AC Jr, Atkins EC: The MAG disabled doctors' program: A two-year review. *J Med Assoc Georgia* 66(10):777–781, 1977.

Tokarz JP, et al: *Beyond Survival.* American Medical Assoc., 535 N. Dearborn Street, Chicago   IL   60610, 1979.

Zitrin A, Klein H: Can psychiatry police itself effectively? The experience of one district branch. *Am J Psychiat* 133(6):653–656, 1976.

II. Case-Finding Problems and Techniques

a'Brook MF, Hailstone JD, McLaughlin EJ: Psychiatric illness in the medical profession. *Br J Psychiat* 113:1013–1023, 1976.

Annas GJ: Who to call when the doctor is sick. *Hastings Center Rep* 8(6):18–20, 1978.

Bittker TE: Why can't we heed a colleague's cry for help? *Med Economics,* Aug. 6, 1979, pp 73–78.

Blachly P: Which MD's are likely candidates for suicide? *Med World News,* April 19, 1968, pp 20–22.

Blachly P, Disher N, Roduner G: Suicide in professional groups. *N Eng J Med* 268:1278–1282, 1963.

Breiner SJ: Early signs of substance abuse by physicians. *Bull—Oakland Co Med Soc* 53(11):7, 1979.

Breiner SJ: The impaired physician—early case finding (therapist survey). *Bull—Oakland Co Med Soc* 53(7):13–14, 1979.

Edwards G: The alcoholic doctor (a case of neglect). *Lancet*, Dec. 27, 1975, pp 1297–1298.

Epstein LC, Thomas CB, Shaffer JW, et al: Clinical prediction of physician suicide based on medical student data. *J Nerv Ment Dis* 156(1):19–29, 1973.

Kales LD, Marten ED, Soldatos CR: Office counseling, emotional problems of physicians and their families. *Penn Med* 81(12):14–16, 1978.

Korcok M: Addiction among physicians: The problems may not be what you think. *Can Med Assoc J* 117(1):89–90, 1977.

Kosbab P: Suicide prevention in physicians. *New Phys* 21(1):21–23, 1972.

Lisansky ET: Why physicians avoid early diagnosis of alcoholism. *N Y State J Med* 75(10):1788–1792, 1975.

Luy MM: How you can spot—and help—your troubled colleague. *Modern Med* 44(4):28–32, 1976.

Parness WD: A doctor-to-doctor hotline you can help start yourself. *Phys Management* 17(11):53–61, 1977.

Pfifferling J: Colleagues should aid impaired physicians. *Texas Osteopathic J* 38(1):8–10, 1980.

Scarborough LF: Mirror, mirror on the wall, who needs help the most of all? *Texas Med* 70:144, Sept. 1974.

Whieldon D: Drinkers, addicts, depressives: What happens when they're doctors? *Practical Psychol Phys* 4(11):13–25, 1977.

III. Medical Training Opportunity for Prevention and Rehabilitation

Adsett, C: Psychological health of medical students in relation to the medical education process. *J Med Educ* 43:728–734, 1968.

Borsay MA, Leff AM: Physician drug addiction: A challenge to medical educators. *Ohio State Med J* 43(11):740–742, 1977.

Cody, J: The M.D.eity: Some personality vulnerabilities of physicians. *J Kans Med Soc* 79(11):605–607, 1978.

Coste C: Resident impairment: The risky business of becoming a doctor. *New Phys* 27(4):28–31, 1978.

Crammer JL: Psychosis in young doctors. *Bri Med J* 1:560–561, 1978.

Crowther B, Felkner L, McDaniel O: Differences among medical professionals in their attitudes toward drugs. *Int J Addictions* 12(1):43–52, 1977.

Dalton MS, Duncan DW: Physician heal thyself. *Med J Aust* 2(9):406–407, 1978.

DeArmond M: Stress among medical students. *Ariz Med* 37(3):167–169, 1980.

Everson RB, Fraumeni JF Jr: Mortality among medical students and young physicians. *J Med Educ* 50(8):809–812, 1975.

Garell DC: Some reflections on physicians' well-being. *New Phys* 27(4):32–33, 1978.

Garetz FK, Raths ON, Morse RH: The disturbed and the disturbing psychiatric resident. *Arch Gen Psychiat* 33(4):446–450, 1976.

Hadley G, Chrispens JE: Unprofessional physicians—some correlative data. *West J Med* 128(1):85–88, 1978.

Kelly, WA Jr: Suicide and psychiatric education. *Am J Psychiat* 130(4):463–468, 1973.

Kligfeld M, Hoffman KI: Medical student attitude toward seeking professional psychological help. *J Med Educ* 54:617, 1979.

Krakowski AJ: Doctor-doctor relationship: III. A study of feelings influencing the vocation and its tasks. *Psychosomatics* 14:156–161, May/June 1973.

Little RB: Hazards of drug dependency among physicians. *JAMA* 218(10):1533–1535, 1971.

Mendlewicz J, Wilmotte J: Suicide by physicians. *Am J Psychiat* 128(3):364–365, 1971.

Meredith RL, Bair SL: Medical students at risk: Evaluation and intervention using a multimodal conceptual model. *Psychiat Opinion,* May 1978, p 41.

Nadelson CC, Notman MT: Adaptation to stress in physicians, in Shapiro EC, Lowenstein LM (eds): *Becoming a Physician: Devlopment of Values and Attitudes in Medicine.* Cambridge, Mass, Ballinger Publishing Co., 1979.

Pasnau RO, Russell AT: Psychiatric resident suicide: An analysis of five cases. *Am J Psychiat* 132(4):402–406, 1975.

Pearson MM: Occupational health hazards of physicians. *Philadelphia Med* 72(2):61, 1976.

Pitts FN Jr, Schuller AB, Rich CL, et al: Suicide among U.S. women physicians, 1967–1972. *Am J Psychiat* 136(5):694–696, 1979.

Rochford J, Grant I, LaVigne G: Medical students and drugs: Further neuropsychological and use pattern considerations. *Int J Addictions* 12(8):1057–1065, 1977.

Russell AT, Pasnau RO, Taintor ZC: Emotional problems of residents in psychiatry. *Am J Psychiat* 132(3):263–267, 1975.

Sacks MH, Frosch WA, Kesselman M, et al: Psychiatric problems in third-year medical students. *Am J Psychiat* 137(7):822–825, 1980.

Scheiber SC: The medical school admissions committee: A preventive psychiatric responsibility. *Psychiat Forum,* Spring 1976, p 16.

Stress common to medical school students. *Psychiat Digest* 38(2):16, 1977.

Thomas CB: Suicide among us: Can we learn to prevent it? *Johns Hopkins Med J* 125(5):276–285, 1969.

Thomas CB: Suicide among us: Habits of nervous tension as potential predictors. *Johns Hopkins Med J* 129(4):190–201, 1971.

Thomas CB: What becomes of medical students: The dark side. *Johns Hopkins Med J* 138(5):185–195, 1976.

Thomas RB, Luber SA, Smith JA: A survey of alcohol and drug use in medical students. *Dis Nerv System* 38(1):41–43, 1977.

Valko RJ, Clayton PJ: Depression in internship. *Dis Nerv System* 36:26–29, 1975.

Vincent MO, Robinson EA, Latt L: Physicians as patients: private psychiatric hospital experience. *Can Med Assoc J* 100(9): see esp. pp 409–410, 1969.

Watterson DJ: Psychiatric illness in the medical profession: Incidence in relation to sex and field of practice. *Can Med Assoc J* 115(4):311–317, 1976.

Yager J: A survival guide for psychiatric residents. *Arch Gen Psychiat* 30(4):494–499, 1974.

Yager J, Hubert D: Stress and coping in psychiatric residents. *Psychiat Opinion* 16(4):21–24, 1979.

IV. Treatment Techniques and Problems

After Hours. *Med Economics* (special issue), Oct. 1, 1979.

Ayres PR: The physician alcoholic: Arch to recovery. *Ohio State Med J* 43(11):737–739, 1977.

Bissell L, Mooney AJ: The special problem of the alcoholic physician. *Med Times* 103(6):63, 1975.

Bissell L, Jones RW: The alcoholic physician: A survey. *Am J Psychiat* 133(10):1142–1146, 1976.

Bittker TE: Reaching out to the depressed physician. *JAMA* 236(15):1713–1716, 1976.

Blachly PH, Disher W, Roduner G: Suicide by physicians. *Bull Suicidology,* National Institute of Mental Health, Washington, DC, U.S. Gov't Printing Office, 1968.

Burrows GD: Stress and distress in middle age—the mental health of doctors. *Aust Fam Phys* 5(9):1203–1210, 1976.

Burrows T: Doctors are people: Stress and medical profession: Part I. *Can Doctor* 46(2):36–46, 1980.

Burrows T: Helping the impaired physician: Stress and the medical profession: Part II. *Can Doctor* 46(3):76–82, 1980.

Burrows T: Managing stress: Stress and the medical profession: Part III. *Can Doctor* 46(4):57–67, 1980.

Connelly JC: The alcoholic physician. *J Kans Med Soc* 79(11):601–604, 1978.

Craig G, Pitts EN Jr: Suicide by physicians. *Dis Nerv System* 29(11):763, 1968.

Crawshaw R, Bruce JA, Eraker PL, et al: An epidemic of suicide among physicians on probation. *JAMA* 243(19):1915–1917, 1980.

Doctors and depression, editorial. *J Kentucky Med Assoc* 78(2):93, 1980.

Dorsey ER: Mental disorders among physicians. *Ohio State Med J* 43(11):744, 1977.

Duffy JC, Litin EM: Psychiatric morbidity of physicians. *JAMA* 189(13):989–992, 1964.

Duffy JC, Litin EM: *The Emotional Health of Physicians.* Springfield, Ill, Charles C Thomas, 1967.

Ellard J: The disease of being a doctor. *Med J Aust* 2(9):318–323, 1974.

Finseth K: Suicide among women physicians (letter). *JAMA* 237(16):1693, 1977.

Franklin RA: One hundred doctors at the retreat (a contribution to the subject of mental disorder in the medical profession). *Br J Psychiat* 131:11–14, 1977.

Freeman W: Psychiatrists who kill themselves: A study of suicide. *Am J Psychiat* 124(6):846–847, 1967.

Glatt MM: The alcoholic doctor (letter). *Lancet* 1(7952):196, 1976.

Goby MJ, Bradley NJ, Bespalec DA: Physicians treated for alcoholism: A follow-up study. *Alc: Clin Exp Res* 3(2):121–124, 1979.

Green RC, Carroll GJ, Buxton WD: *The Care and Management of the Sick and Incompetent Physician.* Springfield, Ill, Charles C Thomas, 1978.

Hall RCW, Stickney SK, Popkin MK: Physician drug abuser. *J Nerv Ment Dis* 166(11):787–793, 1978.

Helping the impaired physician. *Internist* 21(4):3–16, 1980.

Henry S: Alcohol and drugs: The doctor's own prescription (Canadian impaired physician programs). *Can Med Assoc J* 120(8):989–996, 1979.

Herrington RE: The impaired physician—recognition, diagnosis, and treatment. *Wisc Med J* 78:21–23, March 1979.

Hussey HH: Suicide among physicians, editorial. *JAMA* 228(9):1149–1150, 1974.

I'm a doctor—and a drug addict. *Med Economics,* Feb. 18, 1980, pp 85–91.

Jones RE: A study of 100 physician psychiatric inpatients. *Am J Psychiat* 134(10):1119–1123, 1977.

Krystal H, Raskin HA: *Drug Dependence—Aspects of Ego Functions.* Detroit, Mich, Wayne State University Press, 1970.

Leff AM: Medical management of narcotic-addicted physicians. *Ohio State Med J* 43(11)757–759, 1977.

Lemere F: Alcohol and drug addiction in physicians. *Northwest Med* 64(3):196–198, 1965.

Lipp MR, Benson SG: Physician use of marijuana, alcohol, and tobacco. *Am J Psychiat* 129(5):612–616, 1972.

Litman RE: Suicide of physicians: Why does it happen and can it be prevented? *Modern Med* 42(11):34, 1974.

Miller TR: My life as an alcoholic doctor. *Med Economics,* Dec. 12, 1977, pp 192–208.

MJM: One impaired physician's story. *Mich Med* 78(29):529, 1979.

Modlin HC, Montes A: A narcotic addiction in physicians. *Am J Psychiat* 121:358–365, 1964.

Murray RM: Psychiatric illness in doctors. *Lancet* 1(7868):1211–1213, 1974.

Murray RM: Alcoholism amongst male doctors in Scotland. *Lancet* 2(7988):729–731, 1976.

Murray RM: Characteristics and prognosis of alcoholic doctors. *Br Med J* 2(6051):1537–1539, 1976.

Murray RM: Psychiatric illness in male doctors and controls: An analysis of Scottish hospitals inpatient data. *Br J Psychiat* 131:11–14, July 1977.

Murray RM: The alcoholic doctor *Br J Hosp Med* 18(2):144–149, 1977.

Pitts FN, Schuller AB, Rich CL, et al: Suicide among U.S. women physicians. *Am J Psychiat* 136(5):694–696, 1979.

Putman PL, Ellinwood EH Jr: Narcotic addiction among physicians: A ten year follow-up. *Am J Psychiat* 122(7):745–748, 1966.

Renshaw, DC: Physician heal thyself. *Aust Fam Phys* 6(6):598–601, 1977.

Rich CL, Pitts FN: Suicide by psychiatrists: A study of medical specialists among 18,730 consecutive physician deaths during a five-year period, 1967–72. *J Clin Psychiat* 41(8):261–263, 1980.

Rose KD, Rosow I: Physicians who kill themselves. *Arch Gen Psychiat* 29(6):800–805, 1973.

Rosen DH: Physician, heal thyself. *Clin Med* 80(2):25–27, 1973.

Rosen DH: Suicide rates among psychiatrists. *JAMA* 224(2):246–247, 1973.

Rosenberg CL: Doctor rehabilitation: It is working. *Med Economics*, Nov. 26, 1979, pp 114–122.

Ross M: Suicide among physicians: A psychological study. *Dis Nerv System* 34(3):145–150, 1973.

Ross M: Physician suicide risk: Practical recognition and management. *Southern Med J* 68(6):669–702, 1975.

Sargent DA: Treating the impaired physician (letter). *Am J Psychiat* 135(12):1573–1574, 1978.

Sargent DA, Jensen VW, Petty TA, et al: Preventing physician suicide (the role of family, colleagues, and organized medicine). *JAMA* 327(2):143–145, 1977.

Scheiber SC: Emotional problems of physicians: I. Nature and extent of problems. *Ariz Med* 34(4):323–324, 1977.

Seixas FA: The physician with alcoholism. *J Med Assoc Georgia* 65:82–83, March 1976.

Shoemaker KE: Concept of addiction. *J Med Assoc Georgia* 65:84–87, March 1976.

Shapiro ET, Pinsker H, Shale JH III: The mentally ill physician as practitioner. *JAMA* 232(7):725–727, 1975.

Shortt SED: Psychiatric illness in physicians. *Can Med Assoc J* 121(3):283–288, 1979.

Simon W: The suicidal physician. *Minn Med* 55(8):729–732, 1972.

Simon W, Lumry GK: Suicide among physician-patients. *J Nerv Ment Dis* 147(2):105–112, 1968.

Small IF, Small JG, Assue CM, et al: The fate of the mentally ill physician. *Am J Psychiat* 125(10):1333–1342, 1969.

Steindler EM: Help for the alcoholic physician: A seminar. *Alc: Clin Exp Res* 1(2):129, 1977.

Steppacher RC, Mausner JS: Suicide in male and female physicians. *JAMA* 228(3):323–328, 1979.

Suicidal physicians: Problem patients. *Med World News* 17(18):58, 1976.

Talbott GD, Shoemaker KE, Follo ML, et al: Some dynamics of addiction among physicians. *J Med Assoc Georgia* 65:77–81, March 1976.

Vaillant GE, Brighton JR, McArthur C: Physicians use of mood-altering drugs. *N Eng J Med* 282(7):365–370, 1970.

Vaillant GE, Sobowale NC, McArthur C: Some psychologic vulnerabilities of physicians. *N Engl J Med* 287(8):372–375, 1972.

Vincent MO: The doctor's life and practice. *Nova Scotia Med Bull* 50(6):139–142, 1971.

Vincent MO: Female physicians as psychiatric patients. *Can Psychiat Assoc J* 21(7):461–465, 1976.

Vincent MO: Physicians after 65. *Can Med Assoc J* 120:998–1002, April 21, 1979.

Vincent MO, Robinson EA, Latt L: Physicians as patients: Private psychiatric hospital experience. *Can Med Assoc J* 100(9):403–412, 1969.

Vincent MO, Tatham MR: Psychiatric illness in the medical profession. *Can Med Assoc J* 115(4):293–296, 1976.

Von Brauchitsch H: The physician's suicide revisited. *J Nerv Ment Dis* 162:40–45, 1976.

Waring EM: Psychiatric illness in physicians: A review. *Compr Psychiat* 15(6):519–530, 1974.

Waring EM: Medical professionals with emotional illness: A controlled study of the hazards of being a "special patient." *Psychiat J Univ Ottawa* 11(4):161–164, 1977.

What can you do about an impaired physician? *Legal Aspects Med Pract* 8(4):40–49, 1980.

V. Legislation and Law Enforcement

AMA Legislative Department: *State Health Legislation Report,* vol. 3, no. 1, Oct. 1975.

AMA Legislative Department: *State Health Legislation Report,* vol. 4, no. 1, April 1976.

AMA Legislative Department: *State Health Legislation Report,* vol. 5, no. 3, Sept. 1977.

AMA Legislative Department: *Disabled Physician Act.* March 1974.

AMA Legislative Department: *An Act Relating to the Improvement of Medical Discipline.* June 1976.

AMA Legislative Department: *An Act Relating to the Improvement of Medical Discipline: To Require Hospitals, Medical Societies, and Insurers to Report Certain Information Relating to Medical Incompetence; and to Provide for the Maintenance of Records Regarding Medical Incompetence.* June 1976.

Are those tougher doctor-policing laws really working? *Med Economics,* April 2, 1979, pp 106–142.

Berman JI: Legal mechanisms for dealing with the disabled physician in Maryland: Partnership between the medical society and the state commission on medical discipline. *Maryland State Med J* Feb. 1976.

Chart indicating the composition of and disciplinary authority of the state medical practice boards, June 1, 1976. Available from Office of the General Counsel, American Medical Association.

DeMoisey JF: When the bad apples get barreled. *J Kentucky Med Assoc* 78(1):42–44, 1980.

Goldsmith DN, Robertson WO: Medical discipline—a new direction. *Registrant Facts* (Drug Enforcement Administration, U.S. Dept. of Justice), 6(1):4–7, 1980.

Gordon A: Growing pressure to act against incompetent doctors. *Phys Management* 15(2):56, 1975.

Green RC Jr: Virginia's Board of Medicine acts to insure physician competency. *Virg Med Monthly* 103:515, July 1976.

Green RC Jr, Carroll GJ, Buxton WD: Drug addiction among physicians (the Virginia experience). *JAMA* 236(12):1372–1375, 1976.

Hirsh HL: Medicolegal implications of the incompetent, errant, and "sick" physician: Changing times. *Southern Med J* 70(4):421–425, 1977.

Huff JW, Carlton E: The disabled physician in Georgia. *J Med Assoc Georgia* 65:94–96, March 1976.

Lee WJ, Jacobson LA: The role of the Ohio State Medical Board in the case of an impaired physician. *Ohio State Med J* 43(11):760–761, 1977.

Medical discipline: Dealing with physicians who are unscrupulous, disabled, and/or incompetent. A symposium. *N Y State J Med* 79(7):1018–1035, 1979.

Regardie AG: If unprofessional conduct is charged by the California Board of Medical Quality Assurance (medical jurisprudence). *Western J Med* 127:438–441, Nov. 1977.

Smith RJ: The boards and rehabilitation of impaired physicians. *Federation Bull* 66(9):259–265, 1979.

Spies F, Houston A: Medicine and the law: Medical staff liability for the acts of an incompetent physician. *J Ark Med Soc* 75(8):283–284, 1979.

Turner RK: The physician addict: Law, licensure, and rehabilitation. *Federation Bull* 56(6):142–148, 1969.

Ulwelling JJ: The board of medical examiners: A changing role. *Federation Bull* 66(5):134–136, 1979.

VI. Problems of Competence and Ethics

Are tougher laws the answer in correcting incompetence? *Hosp Pract* 11(4):111, 1976.

Chase RA: What to do about the incompetent physician? *Federation Bull* 64(6):163-179, 1977.

Coping with incompetence. *Internist* Sept. 1976, p 3.

Felch WC, Halperin AL: Coping with physician incompetence. *N Y State J Med* 79(12):1921–1924, 1979.

Palmer GS, Astler VB: Florida's answer to the problem of professional incompetence. *Hosp Med Staff* 5(4):12–17, 1976.

Vodicka BE: Medical discipline: VI. The offenses. *JAMA* 235(3):302–303, 1976.

Vodicka BE: Medical discipline: VII. The offenses. *JAMA* 235(6):651–652, 1976.

Warren DG: The discipline of physicians. *J Legal Med* 2(5):43–46, 1974.

White FP: Why don't we put senile M.D.'s out of practice? *Med Economics* 46:77–81, Nov. 10, 1969.

VII. The Medical Family

Anthony M: Al-Anon. *JAMA* 238(10):1062–1063, 1977.

Cameron J: Physicians coping alone. *AAFP Reporter*, Jan. 6, 1980, pp 6–7.

Derdeyn AP: The physician's work and marriage. *Int J Psychiat Med* 9(3&4):297–306, 1978–1979.

Evans JL: Psychiatric illness in the physician's wife. *Am J Psychiat* 122(2):159–163, 1965.

Garvey M, Tuason VB: Physician marriages. *J Clin Psychiat* 40(3):129–131, 1979.

Harrison, Mrs. WH: Characteristics of physicians and their families: Casefinding problems and techniques. *J Fla Med Assoc* 65(5):351–353, 1978.

Krell R, Miles JE: Marital therapy of couples in which the husband is a physician. *Am J Psychother* 30(2):267–275, 1976.

Lewis JM: The doctor and his marriage. *Texas State J Med* 61:615–619, Aug. 1965.

Lief H, Taubman RE: Doctors and marriage: The special pressures. *Med World News* 18(3):38, 1977.

Maddison D: Stress on the doctor and his family. *Med J Aust* 2(9):315–318, 1974.

McCaffrey JC: Do doctors have to be poor parents? *Behav Med* 5(6):39–43, 1978.

Miles JE, Krell R, Lin TY: The doctor's wife: Mental illness and marital pattern. *Int J Psychiat Med* 6(4):481–487, 1975.

Rose KD, Rosow I: Marital stability among physicians. *Med Aspects Hum Sexuality* 7(6):62, 1973.

Seligmann J, Simons PE: The doctor's wife. *Newsweek*, June 11, 1979, pp. 99–100.

Vincent MO: Doctor and Mrs.—their mental health. *Can Psychiat Assoc J* 14(5):509–515, 1969.

Vincent MO: The doctor's marriage and family. *Nova Scotia Med Bull* 150(6):143–146, 1971.

Vincent MO: The physician's marriage: Mission impossible? *Ontario Med Rev* 44(1):7–10, 1977.

Vincent MO: The physician's retirement. *Ontario Med Rev* 44(7):322–325, 1977.

Wallinga JV: The children of physicians. *Med Times* 102(7):115, 1974.

Index